Multiple Drug Resistant Bacteria

Edited by

Carlos F. Amábile-Cuevas
Fundación LUSARA
Mexico City

Copyright © 2003
Horizon Scientific Press
P.O. Box 1
Wymondham
Norfolk NR18 0EH
England

www.horizonpress.com

British Library Cataloguing-in-Publication Data

A catalogue record for this book is available from the British Library

ISBN:1-898486-45-X

Description or mention of instrumentation, software, or other products in this book does not imply endorsement by the author or publisher. The author and publisher do not assume responsibility for the validity of any products or procedures mentioned or described in this book or for the consequences of their use.

Printed and bound in Great Britain by Antony Rowe Ltd, Chippenham, Wiltshire, UK

Contents

Books of Related Interest

For further information on these books contact:

Horizon Scientific Press
P.O. Box 1, Wymondham
Norfolk
NR18 0EH England

Tel: +44(0)1953-601106
Fax: +44(0)1953-603068
Email: mail@horizonpress.com
Internet: www.horizonpress.com

Our Web site has details of all our books including full chapter abstracts, book reviews, and ordering information:

Contributors

Carlos F. Amábile-Cuevas
Fundación LUSARA
PO Box 102-006
08930 Mexico City
MEXICO
Email: carlos.amabile@lusara.org

Julian Davies
Dept Microbiology and Immunology
University of British Columbia
#300-6174 University Boulevard
Vancouver
B.C. V6T 1Z3
CANADA
Email: jed@interchange.ubc.ca

Bruce Demple
Dept Cancer Cell Biology
Harvard School of Public Health
665 Huntington Avenue
Boston
MA 02115
USA
Email: bdemple@hsph.harvard.edu

Neville Firth
Molecular Biotechnology Program
School of Biological Sciences
Macleay Building A12
University of Sydney
NSW 2006
AUSTRALIA
Email: nfirth@bio.usyd.edu.au

Henry S. Fraimow
University Medicine and Dentistry
of New Jersey
Division of Infectious Diseases
Cooper Medical Center
401 Haddon Avenue
Camden
New Jersey
USA
Email:
fraimow-henry@cooperhealth.edu

Peter Gilbert
Sch Pharm Pharmaceutical Sci
University of Manchester
Oxford Road
Manchester M13 9PL
UK
Email: peter.gilbert@man.ac.uk

Jack A. Heinemann
New Zealand Inst Gene Ecology
University of Canterbury
Private Bag 4800
Christchurch
NEW ZEALAND
Email:
jack.heinemann@canterbury.ac.nz

Andrew McBain
Sch Pharm Pharmaceutical Sci
University of Manchester
Oxford Road
Manchester M13 9PL
UK

Alexander H. Rickard
Sch Pharm Pharmaceutical Sci
University of Manchester
Oxford Road
Manchester M13 9PL
UK

Mark W. Silby
Center for Adaptation Genetics and
Drug Resistance
Tufts University School of Medicine
Boston
MA 02111
USA

From: *Multiple Drug Resistant Bacteria*
Edited by: Carlos F. Amábile-Cuevas

Chapter 1

The Rise of Antibiotic Resistance

Julian Davies and
Carlos F. Amábile-Cuevas

Abstract

Bacterial resistance is, beyond the burden it imposes to public health, a superb example of biological evolution. It is also the consequence of a wide variety of biological, but mostly of non-biological factors: marketing, economics, legislation, and education. Is the acquisition of resistance the only difference between pre-antibiotic era microbes and present-day ones? Several other traits might have been selected during these 60 years. This is not only making our current antibiotic arsenal useless but could be potentially undermining future efforts to control infections through antimicrobial agents. Also, a wide variety of non-antibiotic agents are known to select, co-select, or induce resistance phenotypes. Instead of being a "hospital phenomenon", resistance is perhaps being initially selected by antibiotic use, but then maintained by environmental pressures that we might not even suspect. Furthermore, antibiotic abuse is certainly obeying non-biological conditions. There is an intense economic pressure favoring it, and pharmaceutical companies seem to have lost the interest in the research and development of new antimicrobial drugs. Very few approaches are at hand to deal with infectious diseases in the near future.

The Rise of Antibiotic Resistance

Bacterial resistance to antibiotics is a perfect example of biological evolution in our time – the response of a group of organisms (bacteria) to a catastrophic situation. It is a consequence of the interplay of a variety of biological events that resulted from non-biological forces; marketing, economics, legislation, education and medical practice. A comprehensive description of the big picture is difficult to construct, but it is imperative that we attempt this if we are to be at least partially successful in managing infectious diseases in the coming years. That is, to exercise measures to contain the inexorable increase in resistance to the antibiotics that we have, and to delay the onset of resistance when new antibiotics are introduced.

The massive use of antibiotics in the biosphere in the last half-century has created an environment wherein bacteria have been selected to withstand the toxic effects of antibiotics using combinations of the genetic and biochemical mechanisms described in further chapters. Resistance mechanisms are certainly not the only determinants to have been acquired by bacteria during this period: genes for metabolic functions and virulence factors were carried by the same vectors and transferred and maintained by the selective pressure of antibiotic use; they may even have contributed to gene exchange by providing a selective advantage in some environments.

There are probably many genotypic differences between the bacterial species at the beginning of this period and those at the present time. Some idea of these differences might be revealed by a more extensive genomic analysis of the Murray strains, most of which were isolated during the pre-antibiotic era. How might competence for gene transfer, restriction mechanisms, inherent mutation processes have changed between these periods? From the "selfish gene" point of view, during this time-frame mobile genetic elements could have been more effectively replicated and expressed in different hosts, plasmid incompatibility overcome and plasmids became more versatile vehicles for gene mobilization through the acquisition of transposons and integrons; one has only to examine the complex structure of multiresistant plasmids in *Staphylococcus* to be aware of this. Bacterial species with these enhanced capabilities would, in principle, have higher survival potential. Antibiotics have played significant roles in these evolutionary changes, not the least as mutagens and in selecting for hypermutagenic states leading to the facile evolution of plasmid and chromosomal determinants, such as the formation of extended spectrum β-lactamases and other "improved" resistance genes, such as the aminoglycoside-modifying enzymes. Such behaviour is likely to be happening (or has happened) with the increasing use of the newer quinolone antibiotics.

Clearly, the mobilization and acquisition of resistance genes was only one of the many genotypic and phenotypic changes that occurred. Intrinsic physiological responses of bacteria have been shown to lead to reduced susceptibility to a wide variety of xenobiotics, antibiotics included. This may have been an early step in the development of more significant levels of antibiotic resistance and this aspect of the development of resistance has been inadequately explored. For example, constitutive mutants of *marR* and *soxR* are known to be selected under antibiotic pressure. The consequences of such mutant selection have not been examined; might a strain with a constitutive *soxR* be more virulent as a result of its ability to tolerate the oxidative stress in the macrophage? Another general mechanism of resistance is the formation of biofilms; this is most usually a community activity and one wonders if antibiotic use has selected for strains more efficient in biofilm formation as a form of protection; biofilms are well-characterised sequelae of infection in the lung, as with indwelling devices. Thus the connection between selection for antibiotic resistance and increased ability of a pathogen to colonise has been established. While on the topic of biofilms, this is also an environment that favours horizontal gene transfer. Such a juxtaposition of elements predisposing the development of resistance and pathogenicity is hard to imagine!

The obvious conclusions from what we have described above is that environmental pressures on bacteria will continue to produce more virulent species that are capable of adapting rapidly to new chemical insults and environmental stresses. The implication is that it is likely to become more and more difficult to control bacterial infections, for any length of time, by the use of antibiotics.

One significant component of the "resistance" equation that has become more apparent with increased study is the role of other environmental factors, besides antibiotics, that promote the development and maintenance of antibiotic resistance. We mentioned above the role(s) of counter selection processes. The latter can play roles in selection, co-selection or induction of resistance phenotypes. Such are not restricted to clinical situations; agents from disinfectants to air pollutants can select and maintain antibiotic resistance genotypes; there are likely to be other environmental selective pressures that we cannot yet identify or do not suspect. The role of compensatory mutations that maintain the fitness of resistant strains is now well established. Might there be environmental factors that achieve the same purpose? For example, do nutritional factors or inorganic ions play a role? To complete an understanding of what has happened in the bacterial world in the last half-century, it is essential that environmental "maintenance" factors be factored into the equation. Whatever the reason (and one can think of many) multiple drug resistance is generally the rule and it is rare to find bacterial strains that are resistant to only one antibiotic. This characteristic emphasizes the ubiquity of integrons, plasmids, etc. which acquire and maintain clusters of resistance genes such that selection for one of the components ensures the maintenance of all. Truly the politics of "all for one and one for all" have never been more clearly demonstrated!

A full appreciation of the ability of bacteria to exchange genetic information is gradually becoming apparent. There appears to be no limit to horizontal gene transfer and the concept of a "global genome" is an apt description; bacterial genomes are not fixed entities! It is apparent that if any biochemical function is needed for survival by a bacterial species, the required gene(s) can be acquired from other species (under the appropriate selection pressure). In fact, the circumstances are such that competitiveness within microbial populations may be rare since genetic information (DNA) is such an exchangeable commodity. This makes it all the more difficult for researchers to work out the actual paths of development and dissemination of antibiotic resistance in closed environments, such as hospitals. What are the roles of hospital "commensals" in the development of antibiotic resistant strains? Unfortunately, the current methodology available to microbiologists is not up to the task since most bacterial species cannot be grown on laboratory growth media. The isolation of a strain carrying a transmissible plasmid in a clinical situation represents the last stage in a series of genetic transfer and acquisition events that undoubtedly involve interactions between many different bacteria and a variety of different mobile genetic elements. The process involves communities and is not simply a transfer between two isolated bacterial strains on a petri plate in the lab! Nonetheless, in spite of our ignorance of the process, it should be possible to design procedures that limit genetic exchange between bacteria in clinical situations. The most obvious (and easiest) of these is enhancing the level of hygiene, since it is likely that a significant part of HGT involves third parties in the form of people, instruments, bedding, etc. It is generally believed that antibiotic resistance usually migrates from hospital reservoirs to the community. The increasing isolation of antibiotic resistant strains in the latter makes it imperative that steps be taken to interrupt the various forms of transport of organisms and genes. Obviously, a significant effort to reduce antibiotic selection pressure is critical to any concerted effort to reduce the incidence of untreatable organisms.

Similar and, perhaps, even more severe measures will be required to reduce the incidence of antibiotic resistance in farm animals; this source of bacterial pathogens and resistance plasmids has been demonstrated to jeopardize antibiotic therapy in the human population. It has been argued that we are beyond the point of no return in the build-up of resistant strains, but measures can be taken to limit the traffic and national and international agencies such as WHO, EEC and the FDA have proposed measures to achieve this. These measures have been attacked by the pharmaceutical and agricultural industries as being too draconian, but if we are to limit the most insidious form of natural bioterrorism, these initiatives must be instituted and supported.

In what way can antibiotic abuse be curbed? Some measures are mentioned above and there is now sufficient evidence to support the fact that reducing or eliminating antibiotic usage in the agricultural industry and in human pharmaceutical use does reduce on the incidence of resistant strains (unfortunately, they never disappear, for genetic reasons). Perhaps it is time to recognize that **everyone** is responsible for the scourge of antibiotic resistance; the public, physicians, hospital personnel, veterinarians, etc. as well as the pharmaceutical industry. The answer initially lies in good education; the pharmaceutical industry sells antibiotics because people want them. It is clear that the consumer bears a large measure of the responsibility and only a full awareness of the problem and its circumstances is likely to change the situation.

The press and TV could take a more responsible approach in trying to inform their readers rather than trying to scare them. Of course, the latter tactic sells newspapers, so how can one expect an appropriate level of (responsible) behaviour? Does the solution lie in governmental or economic control? These do not seem to be practical solutions since we have been in the antibiotic age for more than 50 years and clinical infectious disease treatment is now completely dependent on the use of antibiotics; this practice cannot be discarded unless reliable alternatives are presented which seems unlikely at the moment. The treatment of infectious diseases requires a constant supply of novel antimicrobials and it is to be hoped that the pharmaceutical industry will support this need. Can this be counted on? It is regrettable that some companies have begun to reduce their research efforts in the area of infectious disease treatment, particularly with respect to diseases affecting developing nations. The charitable organization "Medicins san Frontieres" reports that there is significant marketing pressure in the industry to provide quality-of-life drugs such as the "treatment" of impotency or obesity, in preference to finding effective new antimicrobials. How can the constant threat of infectious diseases be ignored in such a capitalistic fashion?

Fortunately, smaller biopharmaceutical companies have not given up and there are strong efforts to meet the need for new drugs from many companies. There have been significant advances in the identification and characterisation of potentially new biochemical targets, and coupled with new technology in structural chemistry and structure-activity analysis, the probability of discovering novel antimicrobials is being improved. However, this optimism must be balanced with the enormous costs of drug development (in the range of $300 million for each new antibiotic) and the severe requirements of the regulatory authorities. Is it possible that the demand for compounds active against multi-resistant strains will be required so urgently that some antibiotics will be introduced as orphan drugs, in much the same way that AIDS drugs came into being? It is to be hoped that such measures will not be necessary, but some acceleration and "softening" of the clinical and regulatory requirements for antimicrobials may well be necessary. It takes some 12-15 years to take an antibiotic from discovery to clinical introduction (a far cry from the situation in the 1940s and 1950s when antibiotics like streptomycin were in clinical use only 2-3 years after their discovery). Given that high throughput screening, combinatorial chemistry and genomics approaches have not yet provided many new compounds in advanced clinical trials, other approaches are essential.

What alternative approaches that will meet nearer term requirements? Antibacterial vaccines are difficult to develop, although there have been success. Phage therapy is a possibility but it is unlikely to have more than limited applicability to human disease; this approach is thwart with problems of production control and regulatory issues. Drugs targeting virulence functions are an attractive intellectual concept but will they be accepted by the medical profession, and how can their efficacy in treatment be monitored by clinical microbiologists? As has been stated many times by others and now reiterated here, better use of the compounds currently at our disposal, augmented from time to time with the introduction of derivatives with improved characteristics and occasionally novel chemical entities (only one since 1980) appears to be the only way ahead at the moment. But in the face of emerging and re-emerging pathogens, the answer is in our hands: wash them!

From: *Multiple Drug Resistant Bacteria*
Edited by: Carlos F. Amábile-Cuevas

Chapter 2

Gathering of Resistance Genes in Gram-Negative Bacteria: An Overview

Carlos F. Amábile-Cuevas

Abstract

In clinically-relevant gram-negative bacteria, antibiotic resistance genes have been maintained from early gram-negative antibiotic-producing bacteria, or horizontally transferred from other types of antibiotic-producing organisms; also, mutations can generate resistance phenotypes. Resistance genes, most likely originating in chromosomes, gained increased mobility by their translocation to plasmids, that can be conjugatively transferred between a wide variety of organisms. The mechanisms enabling the inter-cellular and inter-molecular mobilization of resistance genes also gave rise to the accumulation of resistance determinants, first within a single cell, then within a single genetic element. Along with the direct clinical consequences of this accumulation, multi-resistance plasmids are now maintained by a variety of selective pressures, including some non-antibiotics agents, due to linkage and co-selection. As we released copious amounts of antibiotics into the environment, we induced a shift in the evolution of bacteria and their genetic elements that is likely to make it much more diffucult to cope with the negative effects of bacterial growth in the future.

Introduction

A given bacterial cell becomes resistant to a drug through two main mechanisms: (a) the acquisition of a resistance gene; and (b) the activation of regulated resistance mechanisms. Also, a bacterial population may survive the attack of an antibiotic if it is organized as a biofilm, which is often resistant -or persistent- to bactericidal compounds (Amábile-Cuevas, 1993). Regulated resistance and biofilms will be discussed in later chapters; this one is devoted to the acquisition of resistance genes, particularly in gram-negative bacteria. To that end, it is necessary to discuss the possible origin of resistance determinants, and the way they travel through genomes; also, since this book focuses on multi-resistance, the aggregation of resistance genes in single genetic elements and/or single bacterial cells will be reviewed.

Acquisition of Resistance Genes: Where From?

From the Murray collection of pathogenic bacteria isolated before the "antibiotic era", we know that antibiotic resistance amongst clinically relevant organisms was rather unusual (Hughes and Datta, 1983). But, in less than 50 years, resistance became a serious public health problem. Although the sole principles of evolution by natural selection, as Darwin initially depicted them, would had been enough to foresee this growing threat, we were learning about microbial genetics just as the first antibiotics became available (see Figure 1). And a number of bacterial features do not entirely conform to Darwinian evolution. The simple selection of an organism's variety by an environmental pressure can only partially explain the rapid evolution of antibiotic resistance. The inheritance of acquired (genetic) traits, and the selection-drived evolution of sub-cellular entities such as plasmids, are some of the aspects that escape from basic Darwinian postulates.

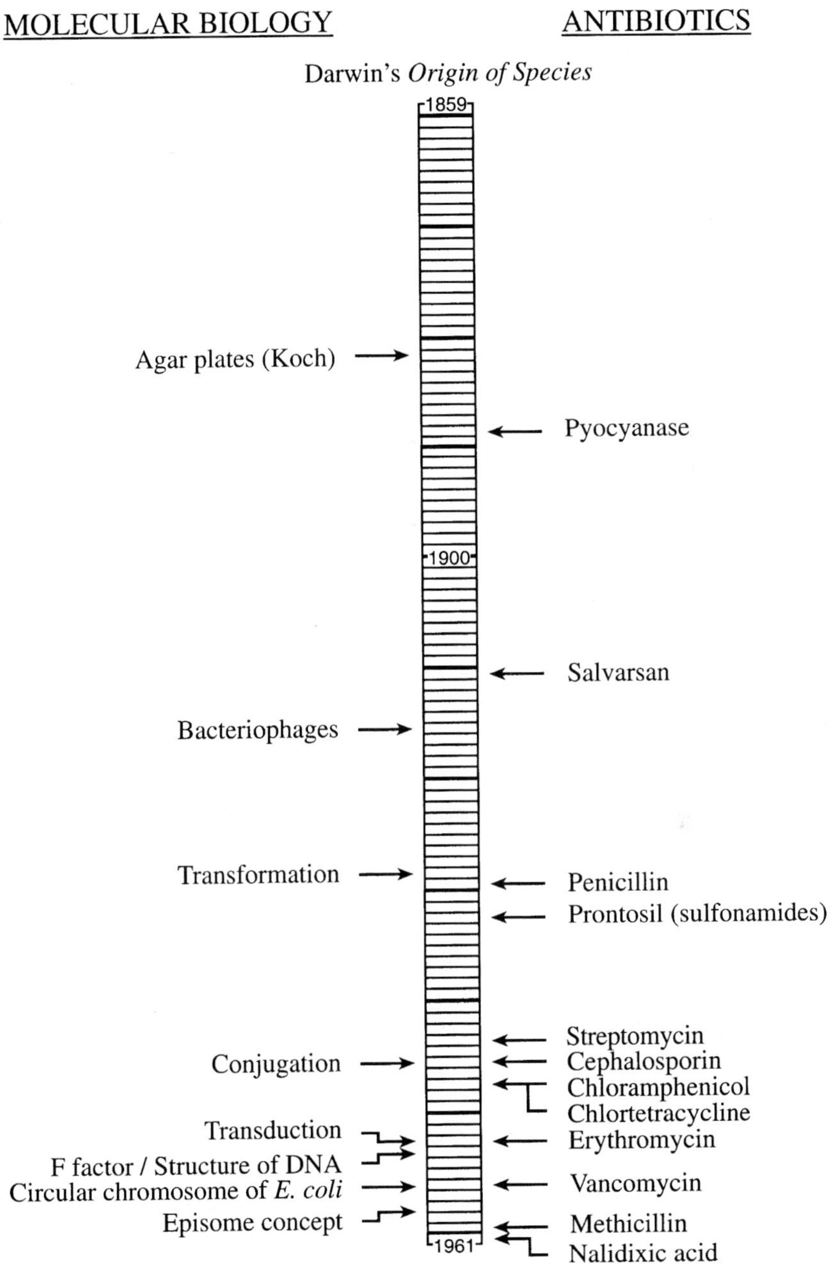

MOLECULAR BIOLOGY   ANTIBIOTICS

Figure 1. Chronology of the "Antibiotic Era" and relevant discoveries in the molecular biology of bacteria. With information from Brock (1990) and Levy (1992). Figure by Isabel Nivón.

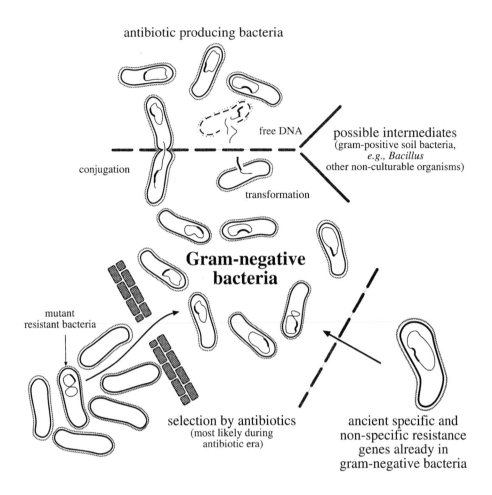

antibiotic producing bacteria

free DNA

possible intermediates
(gram-positive soil bacteria,
e.g., Bacillus
other non-culturable organisms)

conjugation

transformation

**Gram-negative
bacteria**

mutant
resistant bacteria

selection by antibiotics
(most likely during
antibiotic era)

ancient specific and
non-specific resistance
genes already in
gram-negative bacteria

Figure 2. Three possible origins for antibiotic resistance traits (see text). Figure by Isabel Nivón.

    The origins of present-day resistance genes in pathogenic bacteria can be grouped as follows: (a) mutations selected by antibiotics, either some time before their discovery and usage by humans, and then inherited vertically and horizontally, or selected recently by the human use of antibiotics; (b) resistance genes remaining from antibiotic-producing ancestors, such as proposed for chromosomal beta-lactamases in gram-negative bacteria; (c) resistance genes, such as those coding for aminoglycoside-modifying enzymes, acquired from antibiotic-producing organisms, mainly soil bacteria. Figure 2 summarizes these three scenarios.

Mutation

Numbers act in favor of bacteria: they are abundant, and reproduce very quickly. The total number of bacteria inhabiting each human being is approximately 1×10^{13}, and the total number of bacteria in the planet, around 5×10^{30} (Whitman et al., 1998). Also, in very favorable conditions, some bacterial species can duplicate every 20 minutes, achieving a high number of generations in hours or days. Even a very rare phenotype -such as antibiotic resistance- is likely to occur within a bacterial population; and, after selective pressure is applied, this rare organism can rapidly replace the original, mostly susceptible population.

It is highly probable that some of the resistance genes currently spread among bacteria, originated as mutations that were selected by the early use of antimicrobial drugs; or perhaps even before the human use of antibiotics, in environments where trace amounts of these natural compounds have existed for millennia. This initial theoretical framework was used to partially support the use of drug combinations: if a resistant mutant to a single drug arises at a frequency of, for instance, 1×10^{-6}, a bi-resistant mutant would be much less frequent, *i.e.*, 1×10^{-12}, and very unlikely to appear within an infecting bacterial population during therapy. But the rapid rise in the resistance to co-trimoxazole, the combination of sulfamethoxazole and trimethoprim, proved this theory, at the very least, incomplete. Undoubtedly, mutations are the source of many resistance genes of the gram-negative bacteria, such as those encoding modified penicillin-binding proteins (PBPs) or quinolone-insensitive gyrases, but not all of them -perhaps not even most of them- arose as mutations, and they are certainly not restricted to vertical inheritance.

A partial exception to the hereby proposed role of mutations in the acquisition of multi-resistance among gram-negatives is *Pseudomonas aeruginosa*. While carrying multi-resistance plasmids less often than enteric bacteria, mutants that up-regulate the multi-efflux MexAB-OmpM pump can become resistant to beta-lactams, chloramphenicol, fluoroquinolones, macrolides, sulfonamides, tetracycline, trimethoprim and several detergents (Livermore, 2002). In particular clinical conditions, such as when infecting the lungs of cystic fibrosis patients, the bacteria can enter an hyper-mutability state which seems to be responsible for augmented resistance to antibiotics (Oliver et al., 2000). Of course, *P. aeruginosa* can also gain resistance by the lateral acquisition of plasmids, and by phenotypic variation and other phenomena related to biofilm production (Drenkard and Ausubel, 2002).

Persistent Genes

Antibiotics are very ancient molecules, perhaps as old as life itself (Davies, 1990, Davies, 1992). Most antibiotic families, such as aminoglycosides, macrolides, and even beta-lactams (Peñalva et al., 1990), are bacterial metabolites. Although the role of these molecules in the physiology of the producing bacteria is still controversial, it is clear that these organisms bear the genes coding for resistance mechanisms. These antibiotic-producing bacteria, many of them belonging to the *Streptomyces* genus of soil bacteria, harbor genes encoding aminoglycoside- and chloramphenicol-modifying enzymes, for instance. But these soil germs are rarely causative of infectious processes, and are certainly not gram-negatives.

Genes very similar to those in *Streptomyces* spp. have been found in distantly-related organisms, such as *E. coli* and *Pseudomonas* spp. indicating a key role for horizontal gene transfer, in its many forms, in the fast spread of resistance genes from antibiotic-producers to antibiotic-targets (Amábile-Cuevas and Chicurel, 1992). The path of these transfers remains to be ascertained and will be discussed later. But some of the present-day resistance genes, such as the chromosomal beta-lactamase genes in enteric bacteria, may be simply remnants from their ancient predecessors, also antibiotic-producing organisms (Medeiros, 1997). On the other hand, genes governing physiological responses to environmental stress that, when activated, confer a multi-resistance phenotype (mostly due to decreased drug accumulation; see Chapter 4), may have been selected a very long time ago by conditions unrelated to antibiotics. Some of these genes, such as *soxRS*, may have appeared very early in bacterial evolution, residing in gram-negative bacteria long before the human use of antibiotics. Vertical inheritance, associated with the strong selective pressure exerted by the release of antibiotics, can also partially explain the origin of resistance genes in gram-negative pathogens.

Horizontal Transfer From Other Antibiotic-Producing Bacteria

Three main mechanisms of horizontal gene transfer have been described: conjugation, transformation and transduction. The initial mobilization of resistance determinants from antibiotic-producing organisms to clinically-important ones might have relied on the first two mechanisms. Transduction does not seem to represent a major means of transferring antibiotic resistance genes, as it does for the mobilization of pathogenicity islands (Bushman, 2002). Transduction is mostly a narrow-spectrum process and phages in soil, the proposed environment in which original transfers occurred, might not be as abundant as in, for instance, natural waters, where concentrations can be as high as 2×10^8/mL (Bergh *et al.*, 1989). Thus, the likelihood of inter-species phage-mediated gene transfer is probably very low. In any case, more research is needed to clearly ascertain the role of each mobilization mechanism in the spread of resistance genes.

Streptomyces spp., a typical antibiotic-producing genus, and other soil bacteria, such as *Bacillus* spp., achieve transformation competence naturally; *Bacillus* spp. even releases transforming DNA (Lorenz *et al.*, 1991). Several genus of gamma- and beta-proteobacteria are known to also achieve natural transformation competence. The best known examples of clinically-relevant gram-negative germs that can acquire foreign DNA by transformation are *Haemophilus* spp. and *Neisseria* spp. (whose complex nutritional requirements make them unlikely candidates for direct acquisition of DNA from soil bacteria), but some species of the *Vibrio* and *Pseudomonas* genus, as well as the nosocomial-pathogen *Acinetobacter calcoaceticus*, are also naturally transformable (Amábile-Cuevas, 1993). In fact, most enteric bacteria and other gram-negative pathogens seem to have lost the ability to acquire DNA for purposes other than nutrition (Finkel and Kolter, 2001).

Interestingly, *Acinetobacter calcoaceticus* acquire and release DNA for transformational "purposes" (Lorenz *et al.*, 1991); *Pseudomonas aeruginosa*, not known to be naturally transformable, releases DNA for biofilm construction (Whitchurch *et al.*, 2002). Transformation commonly requires a certain degree of homospecificity, making it an unlikely candidate to successfully mobilize genes among distantly-related bacteria. Also, several establishment barriers limit the inheritance of newly acquired genes; these barriers are mainly recombinatorial, with mismatch repair enzymes acting as inhibitors of interspecies recombination (Matic *et al.*, 1995). Nevertheless, transformation is the best-documented pathway for resistance genes to initially mobilize from antibiotic-producing organisms.

Conjugation, which would face many fewer barriers (see below), has been documented from *E. coli* to *Streptomyces lividans*, mediated by a natuarally-occurring plasmid (Gormley and Davies, 1991); but the conjugative transfer from *Streptomyces* to *E. coli* or other gram-negative bacteria has not been documented. Conjugative plasmids are abundant in *Streptomyces*, as are other mobile genetic elements (Rafii and Crawford, 1989). In any case, transformation and conjugation between *Streptomyces* and gram-negatives, directly or through other intermediaries (including an unquantifiable universe of non-culturable bacteria, inhabiting all environments), are the possible initial steps for resistance genes to enter the currently available gram-negative resistance-gene pool.

Although many questions still remain unanswered, these three global scenarios can provide a sufficiently robust framework to understand how gram-negative bacteria gained resistance determinants. But many more questions lie ahead, as we try to explain how these genes mobilize inter-molecularly, and then spread inter-cellularly resulting in the high levels of multi-resistance observed routinely in clinical isolates.

Second Step: Moving Resistance Genes to Plasmids

Transformation may have played a role in transferring resistance genes from antibiotic-producing organisms into the gram-negative gene pool. But a much more active process of mobilization was achieved by conjugation. Aside from the mechanistic differences between these processes, the very nature of the mobilized DNA molecules is particularly relevant: while natural transformation preferentially allows the acquisition of linear fragments of chromosomal DNA, conjugation is usually encoded and mobilize plasmid DNA. Therefore, the second step in making resistance genes capable of wide-range transfers would be to locate them in plasmids. As will be discussed in Chapter 7, the residence of resistance genes in plasmids might have also caused the evolution of resistance to shift from an organism-based process, to a genetic element-based one, following somewhat different rules.

Conjugative plasmids were abundant among gram-negative bacteria isolated before the antibiotic era, as revealed, once again, by the Murray collection (Hughes and Datta, 1983). A paradox arises from this fact: what is the advantage of being a conjugative donor? Except perhaps for retro-transfer, -the process through which the "donor" cell ends up receiving some genetic material from the "recipient" (a process

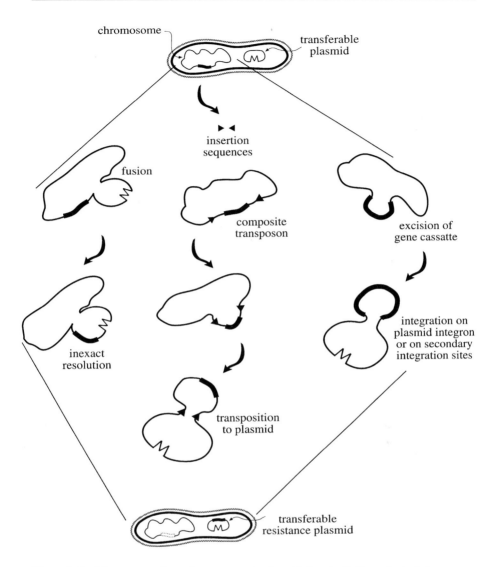

chromosome

transferable plasmid

insertion sequences

fusion

composite transposon

excision of gene cassatte

inexact resolution

integration on plasmid integron or on secondary integration sites

transposition to plasmid

transferable resistance plasmid

Figure 3. Resistance genes from chromosomes to plasmids (see text). Figure by Isabel Nivón.

shown to happen in two steps, instead of during the same conjugative event (Heinemann and Ankenbauer, 1993a), and that occurs even from non-viable cells (Heinemann and Ankenbauer, 1993b))- it is difficult to imagine what a bacterial cell or colony gains by spending energy and other resources to share genetic information, often useful to survive under stressful conditions, with its competing neighbors (Salyers and Amábile-Cuevas, 1997). Again, a likely explanation is that conjugation happens despite bacterial efforts, and that it has been selected as a

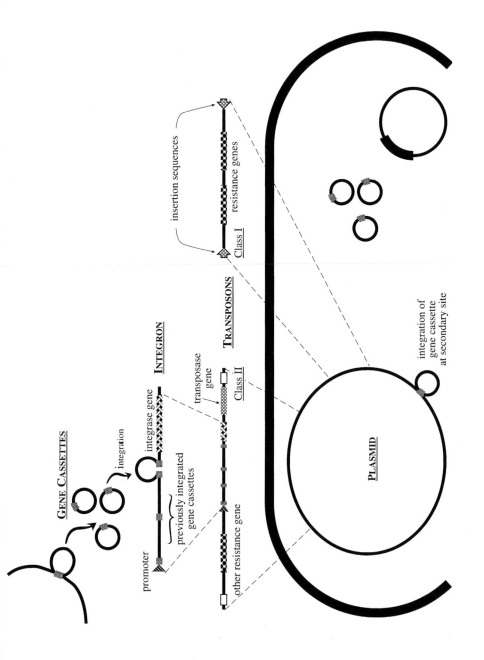

Figure 4. The –updated- matrioshka effect (see text). Figure by Isabel Nivón.

means for spreading plasmids, rather than a means of gene exchange between bacteria. A second paradox is: how did resistance genes get into plasmids? Here I will focus only on the possible mechanisms underlying the mobilization of resistance genes from chromosomes (summarized in Figure 3), where they likely arose, to plasmids. Why this happened is still a very controversial issue, including the question of whether this process was triggered by the human use of antibiotics.

Recombination and the Resistance Plasmid

A number of recombinatorial mechanisms have been identified in bacteria, and some or all may be responsible for the translocation of resistance genes into plasmids. Homologous recombination, as its name implies, requires a high degree of homology between DNA sequences. This kind of recombination is unlikely to target resistance genes, but it is known to create and resolve fusions between plasmids and chromosomes. Because the resolution process may occur at positions different from where the co-integrate was made, some chromosomal genes can be "added" to a previously fused plasmid. The evolution of plasmids seems to rely strongly on this kind of recombination, that commonly yields plasmid multimers; and the fusion of plasmids and chromosomes, as well as their "inexact" excision, was reported almost as early as the existence of plasmids themselves. F' factors, carrying chromosomal segments after integration and "aberrant" excision of F factors in Hfr chromosomes, were crucial for complementation and dominance analyses of mutant genes. The RecBCD pathway of recombination seems to be the major effector of these recombinatorial events (Smith, 1991). Still, these events happen at a very low frequency.

Because it does not require great lengths of homologous sequences, "illegitimate" recombination is a powerful way to mobilize entirely new DNA segments into a plasmid. Early in the 70's, plasmids were shown to act as collections of transposons. Insertion sequences are widely distributed among bacteria; even archeobacteria carry a variety of them (Brügger *et al.*, 2002). These mobile genetic elements accumulate on plasmids due to reasons that are not yet completely understood. Insertion sequences and transposons can mobilize large DNA sequences between non-related molecules, such as chromosomes and plasmids. Some of them carry promoter sequences that enable the expression of genes that lie immediately downstream of the newly inserted mobile genetic element; and some bear promoter sequences that enable the expression of genes within the element itself. Composite, class I transposons, such as Tn*10*, which seem to be DNA fragments flanked by two insertion sequences, provide a nice model for the study of gene mobilization from chromosomes to plasmids, but are not very common in nature.

Integrons, elements containing a variety of resistance genes at specific sites, along with the determinants of site-specific recombination systems responsible for the insertion of those resistance genes, however, are widespread. Integrons are often found in transposons, and have integration sequences, that enable the insertion of gene cassettes (usually a resistance gene; even the most "powerful" resistance genes, such as those encoding carbapenemases are found as gene cassettes in integrons (Poirel *et al.*, 2001), but cassettes encoding traits different from resistance are also common (Collis *et al.*, 2002)). There is also a promoter that allows the expression of the integrated cassette (a powerful promoter, more efficient than the derepressed *tac* promoter (Lévesque *et al.*, 1994)), as well as genes encoding the enzymes required for the insertion and excision of the cassettes; and integrons are mobile elements themselves (Hall *et al.*, 1996).

In this way, circular gene cassettes, one or several, can be inserted into the recombinatorial spot of the integron (alternatively, gene cassettes may be inserted at secondary sites in plasmids and chromosomes (Recchia and Hall, 1995, Recchia *et al.*, 1994)); integrons can be mobilized by their own means or along with the transposon they might be part of; transposons can mobilize themselves between genetic elements co-existing in a cell, such as from the chromosome to a plasmid; and the plasmid can then be mobilized among a wide range of bacterial cells. The matrioshka analogy (Figure 4; Amábile-Cuevas and Chicurel, 1992) actually falls short of capturing the full mobilization potential of this hierarchical system. On the one hand, each element is capable of accommodating several subcomponents (*i.e.*, integrons can carry several cassettes, plasmids can harbor several transposons, and single cells can bear multiple plasmids). More importantly, the system allows the exchange of elements between different hierarchical "sets", something that doesn't work well with Russian doll sets. Integron In53 provides a good example of the complexity that can thus emerge. Harboring cassettes encoding an extended-spectrum beta-lactamase, a rifampin-ADP-ribosylating transferase, a new chloramphenicol resistance enzyme, a multidrug efflux pump of the *qac* family, a novel 6'-N-acetyltransferase, and a fusion of yet another beta-lactamase (*oxa9*) and another aminoglycoside-resistance enzyme (*aadA2*), In53 is itself part of a composite transposon, Tn*2000* (Naas *et al.*, 2001). In any case, following up on the original question regarding how resistance genes came to reside in plasmids, the next logical question is How did resistance genes come to be gene cassettes? That still remains unanswered.

Most studies examining the resistance genes are currently found in plasmids focus on "canonical" resistance genes, such as those coding for antibiotic-inactivating enzymes. The mobilization of such genes into plasmids seems to be a continuous process: chromosomal beta-lactamases from gram-negative bacteria, for instance, are increasingly found in plasmids (Philippon *et al.*, 2002). But other kinds of "resistance" genes have been mobilized into plasmids as well. For instance, the putative product of *tetD*, a gene in the Tn*10* transposon mediating tetracycline resistance, shares homology with SoxS and MarA, regulatory proteins of stress regulons that mediate multiple antibiotic resistance (see Chapter 4). A "mutagenic" plasmid producing quinolone resistance was reported in enteric bacteria some years ago (Ashraf *et al.*, 1991) (the only known example of plasmid-mediated fluoroquinolone resistance in gram-negatives seems to involve target protection (Jacoby and Tran, 2002)). The conjugative machinery itself might provide some resistance towards antibiotics: cells bearing conjugative plasmids can produce biofilms (Ghigo, 2001), that exert a protective action against antibiotics (see Chapter 5).

Third Step: Mobilizing Resistance Plasmids

Conjugation between gram-negative bacteria can be categorized into two groups: typical plasmid-mediated conjugation, and mobilization of conjugative transposons. This second group of mobile genetic elements, very common among gram-positive bacteria and certainly transferable to enterics such as *E. coli*, have mostly been found, in nature, in anaerobic *Bacteroides* spp. among the gram-negatives; they will be discussed later. The role of plasmids, and particularly of plasmid-mediated gene transfer, in biological evolution, has been analyzed elsewhere (Amábile-Cuevas and Chicurel, 1992, Amábile-Cuevas and Chicurel, 1996). Since plasmids –especially conjugative plasmids

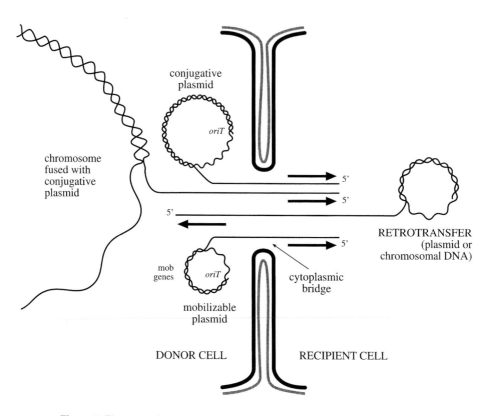

Figure 5. The span of conjugative mobilization (see text). Figure by Isabel Nivón.

(Wolkow *et al.*, 1996)- act as "collections" of other mobile gene elements, and enhance in a number of ways the cell-cell contacts required for gene mobilization, they have extensively contributed to the emergence and spread of resistance genes.

Conjugation allows for wide-range mobilization of genetic information (Figure 5). Mobilizing genes can act *in cis* and *in trans*; therefore, mobile information may reside on the plasmid encoding the conjugative machinery (*i.e.*, the conjugative or self-transmissible plasmid); in a non-self-transmissible but mobilizable co-resident plasmid; in a fused chromosome- or plasmid-plasmid element that is either self-transmissible or mobilizable; or in a chromosomal or plasmid DNA fragment excised by "mistake" after integration and improper excision of any one of the plasmids described above. Also, this mobilization can go forward, from "donor" to "recipient", and backwards, namely by two-step retro-transfer; and may include non-viable bacteria, as discussed before. Conjugation can even bridge the gap between bacteria and eukaryotes (Amábile-Cuevas and Chicurel, 1993), although most likely this is irrelevant to the antibiotic resistance phenomenon. A recent report documents conjugation between bacteria and mammalian cells (Waters, 2001), potentially affecting our own genomes. Originally conceived as a laboratory curiosity, conjugative transfer of multi-resistance within humans and animals has now been demonstrated (Salyers, 1993, Salyers, 1995). Also, the transfer of multi-resistance plasmids in a number of microenviroments, among different bacteria, has been documented (Kruse and Sørum, 1994). A three-page table of reported examples of conjugative transfer in different environments was recently assembled by Bushman (2002).

Conjugative transposons were originally discovered in *Enterococcus faecalis* (Franke and Clewell, 1981), and they are key mobile genetic elements for the gram-positive bacteria. But this kind of transposons, along with a variety of other mobile genetic elements, interacting to gain transferable properties, are not limited to gram-positives –they have also been described in the gram-negative anaerobe *Bacteroides fragilis*. In simple terms, the conjugative transposon excises as a circle from the DNA molecule it resides in, and transfers one of its DNA strands by conjugation to the recipient; afterwards, both circles, in the donor and recipient cells, integrate back into their corresponding host chromosomes.

At a glance, the main difference between conjugative plasmids and conjugative transposons is that the latter are not self-replicating elements, so that they must be integrated into a replicon; otherwise, conjugative transposons can be mobilized among a variety of bacterial genera, bear a number of antibiotic resistance genes, and enable both the *cis* and *trans* mobilization of genetic elements. As a particular feature of *trans* mobilization driven by conjugative transposons, in addition to the mobilization of co-resident plasmids (including plasmids mediating resistance to metronidazole, an anti-anaerobe agent), *Bacteroides* chromosomes often bear an integrated non-replicating unit known as NBU. In a way, NBUs are to conjugative transposons what non-self-transmissible plasmids are to conjugative plasmids: NBUs cannot excise or transfer themselves, but can travel as a result of the *in trans* action of a co-resident conjugative transposon. NBUs display features similar to integrating plasmids of *Streptomyces* spp., and the lambdoid phages. Some of them also carry antibiotic resistance genes.

Yet another distinguishing feature of conjugative transposons, and their associated mobile genetic elements, is that at least one antibiotic, tetracycline, actually induces the mobility of these elements. A 1,000-10,000-fold induction in the self-transfer of conjugative transposons, and a 100-1,000-fold induction in the transfer of NBUs has been reported under low concentrations of tetracycline (and even autoclaved tetracycline, no longer active as antibiotic). It has been proposed that this feature is responsible for the near-100% prevalence of tetracycline resistance among *Bacteroides*, although this phenotype was rather unusual 30 years ago (Salyers and Shoemaker, 1996).

Plasmids and conjugative transposons interact. An extraordinary example of this interaction is the following: a conjugative, R751-derivative plasmid carrying a conventional *Bacteroides* transposon, transferred itself from *E. coli* to *Bacteroides*, where it integrated into the chromosome since it can not replicate in, nor mobilize from, the new host. When a conjugative transposon was introduced into the same cell, however, it transferred the plasmid back to *E. coli*, where it was recovered as a replicating plasmid (Salyers and Shoemaker, 1996). Being the most abundant organisms in the intestinal tract, *Bacteroides* and their mobile genetic elements may contribute a significant degree of mobility to resistance genes.

Assembling Multi-Resistance:
The Selective Pressures

The mobilization of resistance genes, proposed to have occurred originally from chromosomes to plasmids, and then between plasmids, was an important step towards increased transferablity of these traits between different bacterial cells. But it also had a "side-effect": since several of these resistance plasmids may end up in a single cell, and mobile elements can end up in a single plasmid, multi-resistance plasmids can be easily assembled. A multi-resistant strain causing an infection is a much more serious threat than a mono- or bi-resistant one, for obvious reasons. Also, a single conjugative event may allow a recipient bacterium, even during an infectious process, to gain several resistant traits within a few minutes. But the most dangerous aspect of multi-resistance is that it enables co-selection. In this way, a single resistance trait can be stably maintained even without direct selective pressure, as long as there is some selective pressure upon the entire genetic element. This widens the nature of selective pressures maintaining antibiotic resistance in a significant way. The first choices would be antibacterial agents (antibiotics or any kind of toxic xenobiotics) still present and for which resistance genes are carried by the same plasmid. But other maintenance factors that keep plasmids themselves, including those acting before the antibiotic era, can also contribute to the maintainance of resistance genotypes despite the lack of specific antibiotic selective pressures. Since we know very little about how plasmids –especially conjugative plasmids- are maintained in bacterial populations, the design of strategies to control antibiotic resistance is missing vital information. Let's analyze the available clues.

Simple co-selection occurs when a single gene provides more than one advantageous phenotype. *sox-* and *mar-*governed regulons, for instance, protect the bacterial cell against a number of chemical insults, in addition to antibiotics; therefore, any of these insults might act as a selective pressure to keep this genotype. Wide-spectrum resistance enzymes can be maintained by only one of the many antibiotics they protect against (Heinemann *et al.*, 2000). But when resistance genes get linked, together and/or to other kinds of genes, co-selection is much less specific. Some integrons, carry a sulfonamide resistance gene, as a "standard complement", in addition to the integrase system and integrated gene cassettes. Co-selection by antibiotics whose resistance determinants are integrated as gene cassettes in those integrons seems to be responsible for the maintenance of sulfonamide resistance among gram-negative bacteria in Europe, even though the drug hasn't been used for many years (Rådström *et al.*, 1991).

Resistance plasmids and transposons, for instance, often carry antibiotic resistance genes along with heavy-metal resistance genes. It has been proposed (Summers *et al.*, 1993) (and heavily discussed, *e.g.*, Edlund *et al.* (1996)) that mercury released from dental amalgams selects for both mercury- and antibiotic resistance. The common linkage of *mer* genes (encoding mercury resistance, mainly through a mercury reductase that detoxifies the surrounding environment) with antibiotic resistance genes (as in the Tn*21* transposon and its resident integron) has been suggested as the reason for this co-selection. Genes coding for disinfectant-resistance, such as the *qac* genes that protect bacteria from the toxic effects of quaternary ammonium compounds and other disinfectants, are also found in plasmids, linked to antibiotic resistance genes, and mobilized by integrons (Naas *et al.*, 2001).

But natural selections is not shaped solely by killing agents and surviving clones; traits that enhance the fitness of the organism foster the success of the bearer. Virulence genes, that allow the colonization and survival of infecting bacteria, are also found associated with resistance genes in plasmids and other mobile genetic elements. Contemplating the potential for increases in either bacterial virulence or resistance is frightening; but even more disturbing is the realization of their linkage, which can allow the selective pressures acting upon virulence to extend their effects to resistance.

In this way, whichever pressures are selecting and maintaining virulence genes, might also be exerting pressure favoring resistance traits. It has been proposed, for instance, that certain vaccines may increase the virulence of a pathogen (Gandon *et al.*, 2001); although this mathematical model was related to malaria vaccines, similar selection effects might be achieved with anti-bacterial vaccines. At least one vaccine has been implicated in increased bacterial tolerance to an antibiotic, although directly acting upon a permease complex in *Streptococcus pneumoniae* (Novack *et al.*, 1999). Other genes in plasmids, such as those encoding enzymes for the metabolism of unusual carbon sources, could also provide a co-selection framework for resistance, if these two kinds of genes are linked (Heinemann *et al.*, 2000). Since we seldom know what kinds of genes are associated with resistance genes in plasmids, it is difficult to make an educated guess about the potential co-selection pressures.

And Then, All Over Again...

In sum the history of resistance dissemination appears to have proceeded as follows: gram-negative bacteria acquired resistance genes from three main sources, translocated them to plasmids or other mobile genetic elements, and then mobilized these elements, mainly by conjugation, among themselves (and all other bacteria). As several resistance determinants, either chromosomally-borne or residing in one or several plasmids, converged within single cells, the same kind of rearrangements that translocated the first resistance determinants to plasmids allowed the shuffling and assembling of multi-resistance plasmids. Driven by old and new selective pressures, the cycle continues. Multi-resistance plasmids now enter different cells, some times complementing chromosomally-encoded resistance phenotypes, sometimes exchanging determinants to cope with new selective pressures. When we started releasing copious amounts of antibiotics into the environment, we inadvertently set in motion a complex process of evolution whose consequences are so far completely unpredictable. As is the likelihood of reversibility.

Acknowledgments

An ample gratitude is hereby expressed to Marina Chicurel for her very helpful comments.

References

Amábile-Cuevas, C.F. 1993. Origin, evolution and spread of antibiotic resistance genes. RG Landes Co., Austin

Amábile-Cuevas, C.F. and Chicurel, M.E. 1992. Bacterial plasmids and gene flux. Cell 70: 189-199.

Amábile-Cuevas, C.F. and Chicurel, M.E. 1993. Horizontal gene transfer. Am. Sci. 81: 332-341.

Amábile-Cuevas, C.F. and Chicurel, M.E. 1996. A possible role for plasmids in mediating the cell-cell proximity required for gene flux. J. Theor. Biol. 181: 237-243.

Ashraf, M.M., Ahmed, Z.U. and Sack, D.A. 1991. Unusual association of a plasmid with nalidixic acid resistance in an epidemic strain of *Shigella dysenteriae* type I from Asia. Can. J. Microbiol. 37: 59-63.

Bergh, Ø., Børsheim, K.Y., Bratbak, G. and Heldal, M. 1989. High abundance of viruses found in aquatic environments. Nature 340: 467-468.

Brock, T.D. 1990. The emergence of bacterial genetics. Cold Spring Harbor Laboratory Press, Cold Spring Harbor.

Brügger, K., Redder, P., She, Q., Confalonieri, F., Zivanovic, Y. and Garrett, R.A. 2002. Mobile elements in archeal genomes. FEMS Microbiol. Lett. 206: 131-141.

Bushman, F. 2002. Lateral DNA transfer, mechanisms and consequences. Cold Spring Harbor Laboratory, Cold Spring Harbor.

Collis, C.M., Kim, M.-J., Partridge, S.R., Stokes, H.W. and Hall, R.M. 2002. Characterization of the class 3 integron and the site-specific recombination system it determines. J. Bacteriol. 184: 3017-3026.

Davies, J. 1990. What are antibiotics? Archaic functions for modern activities. Mol. Microbiol. 4: 1227-1232.

Davies, J. 1992. Another look at antibiotic resistance. J. Gen. Microbiol. 138: 1553-1559.

Drenkard, E. and Ausubel, F.M. 2002. *Pseudomonas* biofilm formation and antibiotic resistance are linked to phenotypic variation. Nature 416: 740-743.

Edlund, C., Björkman, L., Ekstrand, J., Sandborgh-Englund, G. and Nord, C.E. 1996. Resistance of the normal human microflora to mercury and antimicrobials after exposure to mercury from dental amalgam fillings. Clin. Infect. Dis. 22: 944-950.

Finkel, S.E. and Kolter, R. 2001. DNA as a nutrient: novel role for bacterial competence gene homologs. J. Bacteriol. 183: 6288-6293.

Franke, A.E. and Clewell, D.B. 1981. Evidence for a chromosome-borne resistance transposon (Tn*916*) in *Streptococcus faecalis* that is capable of "conjugal" transfer in the absence of a conjugative plasmid. J. Bacteriol. 145: 494-502.

Gandon, S., Mackinnon, M.J., Nee, S. and Read, A.F. 2001. Imperfect vaccines and the evolution of pathogen virulence. Nature 414: 751-755.

Ghigo, J.-M. 2001. Natural conjugative plasmids induce bacterial biofilm development. Nature 412: 442-445.

Gormley, E.P. and Davies, J. 1991. Transfer of plasmid RSF1010 by conjugation from *Escherichia coli* to *Streptomyces lividans* and *Mycobacterium smegmatis*. J. Bacteriol. 173: 6705-6708.

Hall, R.M., Recchia, G.D., Collis, C.M., Brown, H.J. and Stokes, H.W. 1996. Gene cassettes and integrons: moving antibiotic resistance genes in gram-negative bacteria. In: Antibiotic Resistance: From Molecular Basics To Therapeutic Options. C.F. Amábile-Cuevas, ed. RG Landes/Chapman & Hall, Austin/New York. p. 19-34.

Heinemann, J.A. and Ankenbauer, R.G. 1993a. Retrotransfer in *Escherichia coli* conjugation: bidirectional exchange or *de novo* mating? J. Bacteriol. 175: 583-588.

Heinemann, J.A. and Ankenbauer, R.G. 1993b. Retrotransfer of IncP plasmid R751 from Escherichia coli maxicells: evidence for the genetic sufficiency of self-transferable plasmids for bacterial conjugation. Mol. Microbiol. 10: 57-62.

Heinemann, J.A., Ankenbauer, R.G. and Amábile-Cuevas, C.F. 2000. Do antibiotics maintain antibiotic resistance? Drug Disc. Today 5: 195-204.

Hughes, V.M. and Datta, N. 1983. Conjugative plasmids in bacteria of the "pre-antibiotc" era. Nature 302: 725-726.

Jacoby, G.A. and Tran, J.H. 2002. Mechanism of plasmid-mediated quinolone resistance. Proc. Natl. Acad. Sci. USA 99: 5638-5642.

Kruse, H. and Sørum, H. 1994. Transfer of multiple drug resistance plasmids between bacteria of diverse origins in natural microenvironments. Appl. Environ. Microbiol 60: 4015-4021.

Lévesque, C., Brassard, S., Lapointe, J. and Roy, P.H. 1994. Diversity and relative streghth of tandem promoters for the antibiotic-resistance genes of several integrons. Gene 142: 49-54.

Levy, S.B. 1992. The antibiotic paradox. Plenum Press, New York.

Livermore, D.M. 2002. Multiple mechanisms of antimicrobial resistance in *Pseudomonas aeruginosa*: our worst nightmare? Clin. Infect. Dis. 34: 634-640.

Lorenz, M.G., Gerjets, D. and Wackernagel, W. 1991. Release of transforming plasmid and chromosomal DNA from two cultured soil bacteria. Arch. Microbiol. 156: 319-326.

Matic, I., Rayssiguier, C. and Radman, M. 1995. Interspecies gene exchange in bacteria: the role of SOS and mismatch repair systems in evolution of species. Cell 80: 507-515.

Medeiros, A.A. 1997. Evolution and dissemination of β-lactamases accelerated by generations of β-lactam antibiotics. Clin. Infect. Dis. 24 (suppl. 1): S19-S45.

Naas, T., Mikami, Y., Imai, T., Poirel, L. and Nordmann, P. 2001. Characterization of In53, a class 1 plasmid- and composite transposon-located integron of *Escherichia coli* which carries an unusual array of gene cassettes. J. Bacteriol. 183: 235-249.

Novack, R., Braun, J.S., Charpentier, E. and Toumanen, E. 1999. Penicillin tolerance genes of *Streptococcus pneumoniae*: the ABC-type manganese permease complex Psa. Mol. Microbiol. 29: 1285-1296.

Oliver, A., Cantón, R., Campo, P., Baquero, F. and Blázquez, J. 2000. High frequency of hypermutable *Pseudomonas aeruginosa* in cystic fibrosis lung infection. Science 288: 1251-1253.

Peñalva, M.A., Moya, A., Dopazo, J. and Ramón, D. 1990. Sequences of isopenicilln N synthetase genes suggest horizontal gene transfer from prokaryotes to eukaryotes. Proc. R. Soc. Lond. B 241: 164-169.

Philippon, A., Arlet, G. and Jacoby, G.A. 2002. Plasmid-determined AmpC-type β-lactamases. Antimicrob. Agents Chemother. 46: 1-11.

Poirel, L., Lambert, T., Türkoglü, S., Ronco, E., Gaillard, J.-L. and Nordmann, P. 2001. Characterization of class I integrons from *Pseudomonas aeruginosa* that contain the bla_{VIM-2} carbapenem-hydrolyzing β-lactamase gene and of two novel aminoglycoside resistance gene cassettes. Antimicrob. Agents Chemother. 45: 546-552.

Rådström, P., Swedberg, G. and Sköld, O. 1991. Genetic analyses of sulfonamide resistance and its dissemination in Gram-negative bacteria illustrate new aspects of R plasmid evolution. Antimicrob. Agents Chemother. 35: 1840-1848.

Rafii, F. and Crawford, D.L. 1989. Gene transfer among *Streptomyces*. In: Gene Transfer in the Environment. S.B. Levy and R.V. Miller, eds. McGraw-Hill, New York. p. 309-345

Recchia, G.D. and Hall, R.M. 1995. Plasmid evolution by acquisition of mobile gene cassettes: plasmid pIE723 contains the *aadB* gene cassette precisely inserted at a secondary site in the IncQ plasmid RSF1010. Mol. Microbiol.

Recchia, G.D., Stokes, H.W. and Hall, R.M. 1994. Characterization of specific and secondary recombination sites recognised by the integron DNA integrase. Nucl. Acid Res. 22: 2071-2078.

Salyers, A.A. 1993. Gene transfer in the mammalian intestinal tract. Curr. Op. Biotech. 4: 294-298.

Salyers, A.A. 1995. Antibiotic resistance transfer in the mammalian intestinal tract: implications for human health, food safety and biotechnology. RG Landes/Springer-Verlag, Austin/New York

Salyers, A.A. and Amábile-Cuevas, C.F. 1997. Why are antibiotic resistance genes so resistant to elimination? Antimicrob. Agents Chemother. 41: 2321-2325.

Salyers, A.A. and Shoemaker, N.B. 1996. More than just plasmids: newly discovered gene transfer agents and their implications for controlling the spread of resistance. In: Antibiotic Resistance: From Molecular Basics To Therapeutic Options. C.F. Amábile-Cuevas, ed. RG Landes/Chapman & Hall, Austin/New York. p. 1-18.

Smith, G.R. 1991. Conjugational recombination in *E. coli*: myths and mechanisms. Cell 64: 19-27.

Summers, A.O., Wireman, J., Vimy, M.J., Lorscheider, F.L., Marshall, B., Levy, S.B., Bennett, S. and Billard, L. 1993. Mercury released from dental "silver" fillings provokes and increase in mercury- and antibiotic-resistant bacteria in oral and intestinal floras of primates. Antimicrob. Agents Chemother. 37: 825-834.

Waters, V.L. 2001. Conjugation between bacterial and mammalian cells. Nature Genetics 29: 375-376.

Whitchurch, C.B., Tolker-Nielsen, T., Ragas, P.C. and Mattick, J.S. 2002. Extracellular DNA required for bacterial biofilm formation. Science 295: 1487.

Whitman, W.B., Coleman, D.C. and Wiebe, W.J. 1998. Prokaryotes: the unseen majority. Proc. Natl. Acad. Sci. USA 95: 6578-6583.

Wolkow, C.A., DeBoy, R.T. and Craig, N.L. 1996. Conjugative plasmids are preferred targets for Tn7. Genes Dev. 10: 2145-2157.

From: *Multiple Drug Resistant Bacteria*
Edited by: Carlos F. Amábile-Cuevas

Chapter 3

Evolution of Antimicrobial Multi-Resistance in Gram-Positive Bacteria

Neville Firth

Abstract

The treatment of bacterial infection is increasingly being complicated by the emergence of bacterial strains resistant to a range of agents commonly used to combat them. Among the most problematic in this regard are Gram-positive pathogens such as staphylococci and enterococci. It is now abundantly clear that such organisms possess a toolkit that has allowed them to generate the genetic variation needed to meet the evolutionary challenge that antimicrobial chemotherapy represents. Specifically, through the concerted activities of mobile genetic elements, such as plasmids and transposable elements, and mechanisms of horizontal genetic exchange, these bacteria have assembled arsenals of resistance mechanisms from an extended pool of determinants. Features of specific elements that have played prominent roles in the process will be described, and synergistic interactions between elements will be discussed with due consideration to the significance of selection.

Introduction

Resistance to one or more antimicrobial agents can be an intrinsic property of an organism, as is the case with enterococci, which exhibit significant resistance to a range of agents, including β-lactams, fluoroquinolones and aminoglycosides (Cetinkaya *et al.*, 2000). Alternatively, resistance can arise in a previously susceptible organism either through chromosomal mutation or by the acquisition of pre-existent resistance determinants. Although both strategies have been observed in many bacteria, the relative significance of each differs between genera, presumably as a consequence of differences in lifestyle. For example, in addition to being intrinsically resistant to many antimicrobial agents because of the impermeability of its cell wall (Jarlier and Nikaido, 1994), strains of *Mycobacterium tuberculosis* have developed multidrug resistance to a range of antituberculosis drugs through the accumulation of successive chromosomal mutations (Zhang and Young, 1994; Somoskovi *et al.*, 2001). In contrast, enterococci have supplemented their intrinsic resistance by acquiring new genetic determinants, such as those conferring high-level vancomycin resistance (Cetinkaya *et al.*, 2000).

Although many specific resistance mechanisms have been identified, virtually all can be classified into one of the following three broad strategies. (i) Reduction of cellular concentration; the cellular concentration of an antimicrobial agent is minimised by preventing its passage into the cell through reduced permeability, or by active efflux of it out of the cell. These tactics have been attributed to *fusB*-encoded fusidic acid resistance (Chopra, 1976) and *tetA*(K)-encoded tetracycline resistance (Yamaguchi *et al.*, 1995), in staphylococci, respectively. (ii) Bypass; the action of an antimicrobial agent is either thwarted by over-producing its cellular target, or "side-stepped" by alteration of its target or the recruitment of an insensitive replacement activity. Specific examples include resistance to penicillin conferred by *pbp5* in enterococci (Fontana *et al.*, 1994), tetracycline resistance mediated by *tet*(T) in streptococci (Clermont *et al.*, 1997), and *dfrA*-encoded trimethoprim resistance in staphylococci (Young *et al.*, 1987), respectively. (iii) Inactivation; the antimicrobial agent is inactivated directly by chemical modification or its mode of action is blocked by physical sequestration. *catQ*-encoded chloramphenicol resistance in clostridia (Bannam and Rood, 1991) and *ble*-encoded bleomycin resistance in staphylococci (Sugiyama *et al.*, 1995), respectively, represent relevant examples of such mechanisms. For some antimicrobial agents, it has been found that resistance can arise by several of these strategies. As noted above, resistance to tetracycline can be attributable to distinct mechanisms that result in either alteration of the drug's target site, the ribosome, or active efflux of the drug out of the cell. Similarly, penicillin resistance can alternatively result from overexpression, alteration or substitution of a penicillin-binding protein, or by drug inactivation. In fact, bacterial strains are sometimes found to possess more than one resistance mechanism for the same agent.

The capacity to access existing resistance genes and incorporate them into the genome has been found to underpin the development of antimicrobial resistance, and in particular multi-resistance, in a range of bacterial genera. Indeed, the intransigence of some of the most problematic pathogens is largely attributable to their ability to exploit an extended gene pool, which is afforded by the property of many bacteria to share (donate and receive) genetic material. With the advent of genomics, we are only now starting to appreciate the extent to which horizontal genetic exchange has shaped the evolution of many bacterial genera. In some organisms, significant proportions of the genome, in excess of 20%, possesses sequence features indicative of origins in other hosts (Ochman *et al.*, 2000). Other studies have revealed that in some genera the rates of homologous recombination involving housekeeping genes are significantly greater than previously anticipated (Day *et al.*, 2001; Feil *et al.*, 2001), implying high levels gene flux. Thus, the horizontal transmission of genetic material between bacterial cells is commonplace, there seems to be little or no restriction on the types of genes that can participate, and the evolutionary impact is profound, forming the basis for adaptation to new environmental niches. The survival of bacterial strains in an environment of widespread human antibiotic use represents a salient demonstration of the evolutionary potential of this phenomenon.

For the most part, several decades of research have revealed many more parallels than distinctions between Gram-positive and Gram-negative bacteria in the development of multi-resistance, particularly the involvement of mobile genetic elements. These include plasmids and transposable elements, such as insertion sequences, transposons and conjugative transposons. Similarly, the significance of common mechanisms of genetic exchange, such as transformation, transduction and conjugation, is widely recognized. Notwithstanding these generalities, the specific elements involved and the relative contributions of the various transfer mechanisms differ between organisms. The most notable difference between Gram-negative and Gram-positive bacteria is the widespread involvement in the former of a particular group of mobile elements, the integrons (see Chapter 2). There is currently no evidence suggestive of a significant role for integrons in the evolution of resistance in Gram-positive bacteria. Indeed, apart from a single report (Nesvera *et al.*, 1998), integrons have never been reported in this group, despite extensive studies of a range of genera.

This chapter focuses on the evolution of antimicrobial multi-resistance in Gram-positive bacteria. Since a comprehensive coverage of such a broad subject is not possible in a single chapter, I have chosen to concentrate on some specific well-characterized examples that illustrate a range of broadly relevant concepts, in particular, the nature of associations between resistance determinants and mobile genetic elements, and interactions between mobile genetic elements, which ultimately facilitate the linkage of resistance determinants to form resistance gene clusters capable of horizontal transmission as multi-resistance modules. Such structures pose a serious and ongoing threat to antimicrobial chemotherapy since their involvement in a single DNA transfer event can convert a susceptible cell into a multi-resistant organism.

IS*257* and the Evolution of Multi-Resistance in Staphylococci

The insertion element IS*257*, also sometimes referred to as IS*431*, has been found in numerous genetic contexts in association with a range of resistance genes in clinical isolates of *Staphylococcus aureus* and coagulase-negative staphylococci (CNS)(Table 1). It has similarly been frequently detected in strains of non-human origin. IS*257* is a member of the IS*6* family of insertion sequences, and like other members of this family is thought to undergo non-resolved replicative transposition (Needham *et al.*, 1995; Leelaporn *et al.*, 1996; Mahillon and Chandler,

1998). As a consequence, transposition of IS*257* from one circular DNA molecule (the donor) into another (the target) causes the fusion of the two molecules and the production of an additional copy of IS*257*, such that the resulting cointegrate possesses a single directly-repeated copy of IS*257* located at each of the two junctions between the original molecules (Needham *et al.*, 1995). Additionally, an 8 bp duplication generated at the site of IS*257* insertion is often evident at the extremities of the target molecule. Through this mode of transposition, IS*257* has provided staphylococci a means of inserting one DNA molecule into another. As discussed below, the prevalence of resistance genes found to be flanked by directly repeated copies of IS*257* suggests that this process has been central to evolution of antimicrobial multi-resistance in staphylococci.

Interactions Between IS*257* and Staphylococcal Resistance Plasmids

Clinical staphylococcal isolates commonly contain one or more plasmids. To date, four distinct groups of staphylococcal plasmids have been recognized (Firth and Skurray, 2000). The small rolling-circle (RC) replicating plasmids are usually less than 5 kb in size and can be cryptic or encode one or at most two antimicrobial resistance genes. pSK639 family plasmids range from 8-15 kb in size and encode one or two resistance determinants. Staphylococcal multi-resistance plasmids are usually larger than 15 kb and encode multiple determinants that confer resistance to a range of antimicrobial agents. The largest plasmids from staphylococci that have been characterized are the conjugative plasmids (>40 kb), such as pGO1 and pSK41, which encode a system of around 15 genes that mediate conjugative transfer of the plasmid, and usually carry several resistance determinants. Conjugative plasmids can also facilitate the transfer of other co-resident non-conjugative plasmids. pSK639 family plasmids and some small RC plasmids carry mobilization (*mob*) genes that enable them to transfer using the conjugative apparatus encoded by the conjugative plasmid (Projan and Archer, 1989; Apisiridej *et al.*, 1997).

Other plasmids can be transferred by a process called conduction (Archer and Thomas, 1990; Macrina and Archer, 1993), that involves cointegration into a conjugative plasmid to form a transmissible intermediate that can subsequently resolve to yield the two plasmids in

Table 1. Antimicrobial resistances associated with IS257

Antimicrobial Agent(s)	Resistance gene(s)	Comment(s) [a]	Reference(s)
Aminoglycosides	*aacA-aphD*	IS*257*-flanked truncated Tn*4001*-like element in pSK41 family conjugative multiresistance plasmids	Byrne *et al.*, 1991
	aadD	IS*257*-flanked RC plasmid (pUB110) cointegrate in pSK41 family conjugative multiresistance plasmids	Byrne *et al.*, 1990
		IS*257*-flanked RC plasmid (pUB110) cointegrate in chromosomal SCC*mec* elements; Potential IS*257*-hybrid promoter transcribed resistance gene	Byrne *et al.*, 1991
Antiseptics/Disinfectants	*smr*	IS*257*-flanked RC plasmid in pSK41 family conjugative multiresistance plasmids	Berg *et al.*, 1998
		IS*257*-flanked RC plasmid in pSK639 family plasmids	Leelaporn *et al.*, 1996
β-lactams including methicillin	*mecA*	Derepression of resistance gene due to IS*257*-mediated deletion of *mecI* repressor	Katayama *et al.*, 2001
Bleomycin	*ble*	IS*257*-flanked RC plasmid (pUB110) cointegrate in pSK41 family conjugative multiresistance plasmids	Byrne *et al.*, 1991
		IS*257*-flanked RC plasmid (pUB110) cointegrate in chromosomal SCC *mec* elements	Byrne *et al.*, 1991
Cadmium	*cadD*	IS*257*-flanked RC plasmid cointegrate in unclassified resistance plasmid; Potential IS*257*-hybrid promoter transcribed resistance gene	Crupper *et al.*, 1999; Simpson *et al.*, 2000

Antibiotic	Gene	Description	Reference
Mercury/Organomercurials	merA-merB	IS257-flanked resistance genes in β-lactamase/heavy metal resistance family multiresistance plasmids	Laddaga et al., 1987
		IS257-flanked resistance genes in chromosomal SCCmec elements	Ito et al., 2001
Mupirocin	mupA	IS257-flanked resistance gene in pSK41 family conjugative multiresistance plasmids; potential IS257-hybrid promoter transcribed resistance gene	Morton et al., 1995
Streptogramins (type A)	vat	IS257-flanked plasmid (pAMβ1-like) cointegrate in multiresistance plasmids	Allignet and El Solh, 1999
Tetracycline	tetA(K)	IS257-flanked RC plasmid in pSK639 family plasmids	Leelaporn et al., 1996
		IS257-flanked RC plasmid (pT181) cointegrate in unclassified resistance plasmids	Werckenthin et al., 1996; Needham et al., 1994
		IS257-flanked RC plasmid (pT181) cointegrate in chromosomal SCCmec elements; IS257-hybrid promoter transcribed resistance gene	Simpson et al., 2000
Trimethoprim	dfrA	IS257-flanked resistance gene in pSK639 family plasmids; IS257-hybrid promoter transcribed resistance gene	Leelaporn et al., 1994; Leelaporn et al., 1996
		IS257-flanked pSK639 family plasmid cointegrate in pSK1 family multiresistance plasmids	Leelaporn et al., 1996
		IS257-flanked pSK639 family plasmid cointegrate in pSK41 family conjugative multiresistance plasmids	Berg et al., 1998
Virginiamycin	vgb	IS257-flanked plasmid (pAMβ1-like) cointegrate in multiresistance plasmids	Allignet and El Solh, 1999

a See text for details.

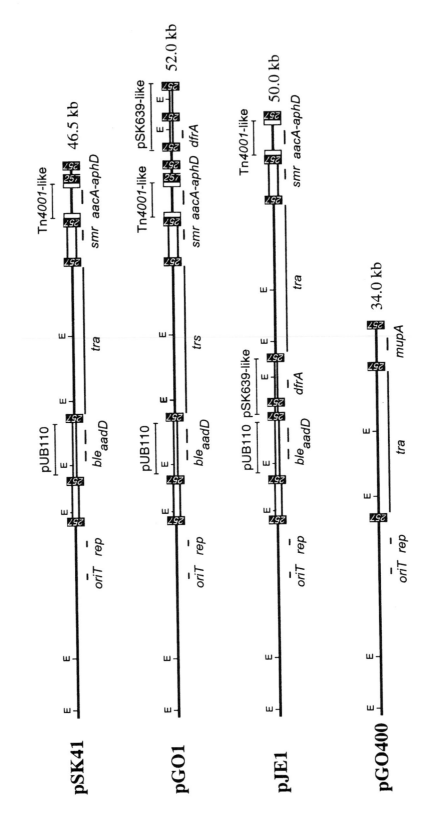

Figure 1. Staphylococcal conjugative multi-resistance plasmids pSK41, pGO1, pJE1 and pGO400 (Evans and Dyke, 1988; Morton *et al.*, 1993; Morton *et al.*, 1995; Berg *et al.*, 1998). Extents of cointegrated pUB110 and pSK639-like plasmids, and truncated Tn*4001*-like elements, are indicated above the maps. Double horizontal lines denote cointegrated plasmids. The positions of IS*257* elements, truncated copies of IS*256* (vertical boxes), and *Eco*RI restriction endonuclease cleavage sites (E) are shown. Loci encoding the following functions are indicated beneath the maps: *aadD/aacA-aphD*, aminoglycoside resistance; *ble*, bleomycin resistance; *dfrA*, trimethoprim resistance; *mupA*, mupirocin resistance; *oriT*, origin of conjugative DNA transfer; *rep*, initiation of plasmid replication; *smr*, multidrug resistance to antiseptics and disinfectants; *tra*, conjugative transfer. Plasmid sizes are indicated on the right.

the recipient. Bacteriophage-mediated transduction and a poorly understood mechanism known variously as mixed culture transfer or phage-mediated conjugation provide additional avenues of lateral gene and plasmid transfer among staphylococci (Lacey, 1980; Lyon and Skurray, 1987). The pSK639 family, multi-resistance, and conjugative plasmids are all believed to utilize theta mode replication (Gering *et al.*, 1996; Apisiridej *et al.*, 1997; Firth *et al.*, 2000). With the exception of pSK639 family plasmids, highly similar if not identical plasmids of each type have been found in strains of *S. aureus* and coagulase-negative staphylococci. This observation is consistent with interspecific plasmid transfer in nature, and such transfer is demonstrable in the laboratory (Forbes and Schaberg, 1983; McDonnell *et al.*, 1983; Thomas and Archer, 1992). In the case of the pSK639 family plasmids, autonomously replicating forms have to date only been identified in *S. epidermidis*, but cointegrated remnants of pSK639-like plasmids have been found in *S. aureus* (Berg *et al.*, 1998; Firth and Skurray, 1998), and plasmids of this type have been shown in the laboratory to replicate in this host. Interactions between IS*257* and each of the staphylococcal plasmid types have been reported. Indeed, with the exception of the small RC plasmids, the carriage of one or more copies of IS*257* appears commonplace for staphylococcal plasmids; size constraints associated with rolling-circle replication appear to effectively preclude the carriage of transposable elements by RC plasmids (Novick, 1989; Helinski *et al.*, 1996).

The conjugative plasmids represent the most striking illustration of the impact of IS*257*, which appears to have shaped the recent evolution of these plasmids in a timeframe presumed to correspond to the widespread use of antimicrobial agents by man. Conjugative plasmids typically contain multiple copies of IS*257*, almost always in direct orientation with respect to each other (Figure 1). For example, pGO1 contains nine directly oriented copies of IS*257* and a single copy in inverted orientation (Morton *et al.*, 1993). Analysis of the complete nucleotide sequence of the 46 kb conjugative plasmid pSK41, which contains seven copies of IS*257*, revealed that five of the directly repeated copies flank three cointegrated RC plasmids. One of these integrated plasmids is identical to pUB110, encoding *aadD* and *ble* genes which confer aminoglycoside and bleomycin resistance, respectively (Sadaie *et al.*, 1980; Semon *et al.*, 1987; Byrne *et al.*, 1991); the second confers resistance to antiseptics and disinfectants via a *smr* (formerly *qacC*) multidrug resistance determinant (Littlejohn *et al.*, 1991); and the third encodes a putative membrane protein of unknown function (Berg *et al.*, 1998). These cointegrated plasmids are believed to have been captured as a result of non-resolved replicative transposition of IS*257* elements carried by a pSK41 precursor into the RC plasmids.

The closely related conjugative plasmids pGO1 and pJE1 are thought to carry one further cointegrated plasmid closely related to pSK639 (see above), mediating trimethoprim resistance via a *dfrA*-encoded S1 trimethoprim-insensitive dihydrofolate reductase (Rouch *et al.*, 1989; Berg *et al.*, 1998). Like the three cointegrated RC plasmids carried by these plasmids described above, incorporation of the pSK639-like plasmid into a pGO1 progenitor is likely to have resulted from IS*257* transposition, although in this case the element responsible might have resided on the pSK639-like plasmid. In contrast, incorporation of a pSK639-like plasmid into a pJE1 precursor appears to have resulted from homologous recombination between IS*257* copies pre-existing on each plasmid (Berg *et al.*, 1998). The replicative nature of IS*257* transposition accounts for the additional copy of IS*257* carried by pGO1, in comparison to pJE1. These examples illustrate the two methods by which IS*257* can mediate the capture of resistance genes; through its mechanism of transposition, and by acting as a portable substrate for homologous recombination. The latter method is likely to be quite significant since recent estimates suggest a high rate of homologous recombination in *S. aureus*, which exceeds the mutation rate (Feil *et al.*, 2001).

For each of the small plasmids carried within pSK41, and presumably pGO1 and pJE1, sequences usually essential for replication of the cointegrated plasmid have been insertionally inactivated by IS*257* in the course of cointegration, and/or deleted as a consequence of subsequent IS*257*–mediated flanking deletions. The replication systems carried by RC and pSK639-like plasmids typically mediate maintenance at copy numbers significantly higher than those of larger multi-resistance and conjugative plasmids. The expression of such replication systems in the context of a large cointegrate plasmid would be expected to elevate the copy number of the plasmid to a level that would be metabolically burdensome to the host cell and hence be detrimental to the survival of both host and plasmid. Disruption of these replication systems therefore effectively represents a prerequisite for assembly of such composite multi-resistance plasmids. Thus, IS257 affords staphylococci not only ways to acquire useful functions such as resistance determinants, but also means of inactivating or deleting non-essential or deleterious DNA sequences. Flanking deletions are an expected outcome of intramolecular transposition of IS257 (Skurray and Firth, 1997; Firth and Skurray, 1998). Deletions have also been observed to occur as a consequence of homologous recombination between IS257 copies on pSK41 (Berg *et al.*, 1998).

pSK41-like plasmids also contain a derivative of the IS256-bounded composite transposon, Tn4001 (Byrne *et al.*, 1990). The central region of this element contains the *aacA-aphD* gene that encodes a bifunctional aminoglycoside-modifying enzyme, AAC(6')-APH(2"), which confers resistance to gentamicin, tobramycin and kanamycin (Rouch *et al.*, 1987). Tn4001-like elements have played a significant role in the emergence and dissemination of aminoglycoside resistance, most notably gentamicin resistance, in staphylococci (Paulsen *et al.*, 1997), enterococci (Hodel-Christian and Murray, 1991), and streptococci (Horaud *et al.*, 1996). The copies of IS256 at both ends of the Tn4001-like elements on pSK41-like plasmids have been truncated as a result of IS257 flanking deletions (Byrne *et al.*, 1990), rendering the element transpositionally defective. By preventing transposition to other plasmids or the chromosome, the immobilization of this transposon has presumably contributed to the evolutionary success of the pSK41-like plasmids by ensuring that aminoglycoside resistance is linked to carriage of the plasmid. This selfish behavior is an example of evolutionary forces operating at the level of plasmids rather than their host.

IS257-flanked cointegrated plasmids are not confined to the conjugative plasmids of staphylococci. Cointegrated RC plasmids encoding *smr* or *tetA*(K) have been characterized in pSK639 family plasmids (Leelaporn *et al.*, 1996), and plasmid cointegrates which confer *vgb*-encoded virginiamycin resistance, *vat*-encoded resistance to streptogramin type A antibiotics (Allignet and El Solh, 1999) and *cadD*-mediated cadmium resistance (Crupper *et al.*, 1999) have been found in staphylococcal multi-resistance plasmids. Other plasmid-encoded

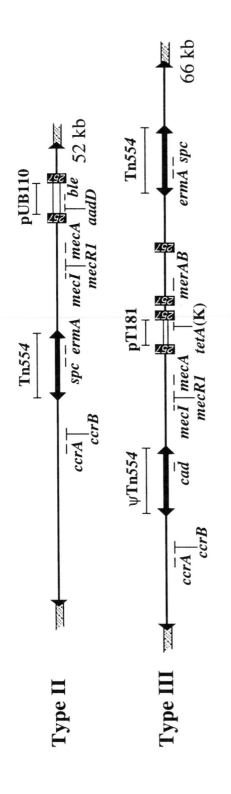

Figure 2. Type II and III staphylococcal SCC*mec* resistance islands (Hiramatsu *et al.*, 2001). Extents of the cointegrated plasmids pUB110 and pT181, and the transposons Tn*554* and ψTn*554*, are indicated above the maps. Terminal inverted repeats of Tn*554* and ψTn*554*, and SCC*mec* elements, are indicated by arrowheads. Double horizontal lines denote cointegrated plasmids, whereas non-SCC*mec* chromosomal DNA is indicated by hatching. The positions of IS*257* copies are indicated beneath the maps. Loci encoding the following functions are indicated beneath the maps: *aadD*, aminoglycoside resistance; *ble*, bleomycin resistance; *cad*, cadmium resistance; *ccrA/ccrB*, cassette chromosome recombinase; *ermA*, MLS resistance; *mecI/mecR1*, regulation of *mecA*; *merAB*, mercury/organomercurial resistance; *spc*, spectinomycin resistance; *tetA*(K), tetracycline resistance. Sizes of the SCC*mec* elements are indicated on the right.

resistance determinants have also been found with flanking copies of IS257, including the mupirocin resistance gene *mupA* (Needham *et al.*, 1994; Morton *et al.*, 1995) and the *merA-merB* operon that confers resistance to mercury/organomercurials (Laddaga *et al.*, 1987). These IS257-flanked determinants are not known to be derived from cointegrated plasmids but this possibility cannot be excluded.

IS257 and Chromosomal SCC*mec* Resistance Islands

IS257 has also been found in the chromosome of staphylococcal isolates. Notably, one or more copies of IS257 appear to be ubiquitous within the region of the chromosome associated with methicillin resistance in methicillin resistant *S. aureus* (MRSA), commonly referred to as the *mec* region (Figure 2). The genetic basis of this *mec* determinant is now known to be a novel family of mobile genetic elements, termed staphylococcal cassette chromosome *mec* (SCC*mec*) (Ito *et al.*, 1999; Katayama *et al.*, 2000; Ito *et al.*, 2001). SCC*mec* contains the *mecA* gene that encodes the low affinity penicillin-binding protein PBP2′ (also referred to as PBP2a) that is responsible for resistance to β-lactam antibiotics including methicillin (Hartman and Tomasz, 1984; Song *et al.*, 1987), and two genes, *ccrA and ccrB*, which mediate site-specific integration and excision of the element into and from a specific chromosomal integration site (Katayama *et al.*, 2000). Ranging from 21-67 kb in size, SCC*mec* can be regarded as a resistance island (Hiramatsu *et al.*, 2001). Current evidence suggests that SCC*mec* elements have been acquired by *S. aureus* on several occasions (Fitzgerald *et al.*, 2001; Hiramatsu *et al.*, 2001), and these elements have also been found in a range of CNS (Katayama *et al.*, 2001). SCC*mec* appears to be restricted to the genus *Staphylococcus* but its origin is not known, although a gene homologous to *mecA* appears to be ubiquitous in *S. sciuri* (Wu *et al.*, 1996; Wu *et al.*, 1998).

Determinants encoding resistance to non-β-lactam agents are also variously found within members of SSC*mec*, including the transposons Tn554, which confers *ermA*-encoded resistance to macrolides, lincosamides and streptogramin type B (MLS) antibiotics (Murphy, 1985b) and *spc*-encoded spectinomycin resistance (Murphy, 1985a), and ψTn554 which confers *cad*-encoded cadmium resistance (Witte *et al.*, 1986; Dubin *et al.*, 1992; Ito *et al.*, 2001). All examples of SCC*mec* characterized to date carry at least one copy of IS257 downstream of the *mecA* gene. These elements have facilitated the incorporation of further resistance genes within SCC*mec* resistance islands, in a manner analogous to that described above for conjugative staphylococcal multi-resistance plasmids. Specifically, SCC*mec* have been found to carry IS*257*-flanked cointegrated copies of the RC plasmids pUB110 (see above) and pT181, the latter conferring tetracycline resistance via an efflux pump encoded by the *tetA*(K) gene (Gillespie *et al.*, 1986; Byrne *et al.*, 1991; Stewart *et al.*, 1994; Oliveira *et al.*, 2000). A *merA-merB* mercury/ organomercurial resistance determinant equivalent to the IS*257*-flanked segment found in some multi-resistance plasmids is also found downstream of *mecA* in some SCC*mec* (Gillespie *et al.*, 1987; Ito *et al.*, 2001).

Involvement of IS*257* in Resistance Gene Expression

The IS*257*-flanked cointegrated copy of pT181 identified within the *mec* region of Australian *S. aureus* isolates illustrates another important property of IS*257*; the capacity to facilitate transcription of adjacent genes (Simpson *et al.*, 2000). A sequence, TTGCAA, with the potential to act as a −35 promoter sequence (consensus TTGACA) is located within the terminal inverted repeat at each end of IS*257*. Insertion of IS*257* adjacent to sequence resembling a −10 promoter sequence (consensus TATAAT) can result in the formation of an IS*257*-hybrid promoter; such −10–like sequences are quite prevalent in staphylococci due to the high A+T content of the genome. In the case of the pT181 cointegrate, IS*257* inserted such that −35 sequence of the promoter normally responsible for transcription of *tetA*(K) in pT181 is replaced by the −35 sequence within the end of the insertion sequence. The resulting IS*257*-hybrid promoter was found to be considerably more powerful than the original. As a consequence, a strain carrying pT181 as a chromosomal-cointegrate is resistant to significantly higher levels of tetracycline than one carrying the autonomous multicopy form of the plasmid. Transcription directed from an IS*257*-hybrid promoter has also been shown to be responsible for widely-disseminated high-level trimethoprim resistance conferred by the *dfrA* gene found on pSK639, multi-resistance and conjugative plasmids in *S. aureus* and CNS (Leelaporn *et al.*, 1994). Other probable IS*257*-hybrid promoters have been identified upstream of the *aadA* aminoglycoside resistance gene encoded by the pUB110 cointegrate carried by some SCC*mec* elements, and the *cadD* and *mupA* genes carried by the plasmids pRW001 and pGO400, which confer cadmium and mupirocin resistance, respectively (Simpson *et al.*, 2000). Additionally, a complete but relatively weak outwardly directed promoter has been identified at one end of IS*257*, raising the possibility that this element might contribute to transcription of adjacent genes in cases where a hybrid promoter is not formed (Simpson *et al.*, 2000).

IS*257* has been shown to be involved directly in the mediation of methicillin resistance in some *S. haemolyticus* strains. In addition to the ubiquitous copy of IS*257* located downstream of *mecA*, SCC*mec* elements found in this species possess an upstream copy of IS*257* (Katayama *et al.*, 2001). In some cases, adjacent deletions mediated by this upstream element extend into and obliterate the genes *mecI* and *mecR1*, which are located immediately upstream of, and transcribed divergently from, *mecA* (Katayama *et al.*, 2001). *mecI* and *mecR1* encode a transcriptional repressor and sensor protein, respectively, which form a regulatory system that facilitates inducible transcription of *mecA* in response to the presence of β-lactams (Niemeyer *et al.*, 1996). The inactivation of *mecI* caused by IS*257*-mediated flanking deletions therefore results in increased levels of *mecA* transcription (Katayama *et al.*, 2001). Such de-repression of *mecA* expression is thought to be a prerequisite for the expression of a methicillin resistant phenotype; in SCC*mec* carried by MRSA, the *mecI* gene is typically found to have been subject to mutation or deletion, the latter associated with the insertion elements IS*1272* and IS*256* (Archer and Niemeyer, 1994; Kobayashi *et al.*, 1998; Sharma *et al.*, 1998; Kobayashi *et al.*, 1999; Oliveira *et al.*, 2000).

In the context of a DNA molecule capable of horizontal transmission, such as mobilisable or conjugative plasmids or SCC*mec* elements, the carriage of IS*257* affords a ready mechanism to collect resistance determinants as the molecule moves horizontally from cell to cell, potentially crossing species and genera boundaries. In such a situation, the horizontally-transmissible molecule is behaving as selfish DNA, its potential for survival enhanced by the fitness advantage it may afford a subsequent host, rather than the host from which the gene was collected. The capacity of IS*257* to mediate the assembly of multi-resistance gene clusters, such as those described above, and in some cases facilitate their transcription, appears to have allowed it to play a role in staphylococci that is reminiscent of the role fulfilled by integrons in a number of Gram-negative genera. Although the mechanisms and substrates involved are distinct, integrase-mediated site-specific recombination involving circular gene cassettes in the case of integrons,

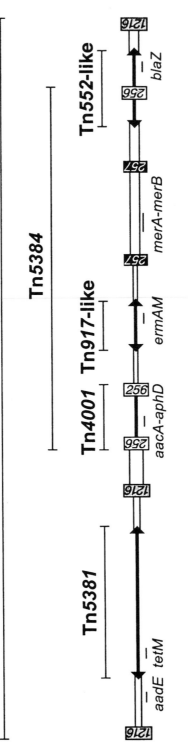

Figure 3. *E. faecalis* transposon Tn*5385* (Rice, 2000). Extents of Tn*5385*, Tn*5384*, Tn*5381*, Tn*4001*, Tn*917*-like and Tn*552*-like transposons, are indicated above the map. Terminal inverted repeats of Tn*5381*, Tn*917*-like and Tn*552*-like transposons are indicated by arrowheads. Double horizontal lines denote cointegrated plasmids. The positions of IS*256*, IS*257* and IS*1216* copies are shown. Loci encoding the following functions are indicated beneath the map: *aadE/aacA-aphD*, aminoglycoside resistance; *blaZ*, β-lactam resistance; *ermAM*, resistance to streptogramin type B antibiotics; *merA-merB*, mercury/organomercurial resistance; *tetM*, tetracycline and minocycline resistance.

as opposed to non-resolved replicative transposition involving circular plasmids, most commonly RC plasmids, in the case of IS*257*, the net result, the capture and clustering of resistance genes, is equivalent.

Multi-Resistance Element Tn*5385* From *Enterococcus faecalis*

A spectacular example of clustering of resistance determinants, and the mobile genetic elements with which they are associated, is Tn*5385* (Rice and Carias, 1998; Rice, 2000), identified in the chromosome of a clinical *E. faecalis* strain (Bonafede *et al.*, 1997). This composite transposon-like structure is approximately 65 kb in size and is bounded by directly-repeated copies of the enterococcal insertion element IS*1216* (Rice and Carias, 1998); like IS*257* described above, IS*1216* is a member of the IS*6* family of insertion sequences (Mahillon and Chandler, 1998). As illustrated diagrammatically in Figure 3, Tn*5385* contains a third directly-repeated copy of IS*1216*, three copies of IS*256* (see above), which is prevalent in both staphylococci (Lyon *et al.*, 1987; Dyke *et al.*, 1992) and enterococci (Rice and Thorisdottir, 1994), in both direct and inverted orientations, and two directly-repeated copies of IS*257*. At least five other transposons, and remnants of at least 4 plasmids, appear to be encompassed within Tn*5385*. The entire assemblage contains six antimicrobial resistance determinants.

Adjacent to and truncated by the leftmost copy of IS*1216* in Tn*5385* is an open reading frame that is nearly identical to a gene carried by a plasmid from *Streptococcus pyogenes* (Rice and Carias, 1998). To the right of this plasmid remnant is an *aadE* aminoglycoside adenyl-transferase gene that confers high-level streptomycin resistance (Rice and Carias, 1998). Between *aadE* and the internal copy of IS*1216* is the Tn*916*-like conjugative transposon, Tn*5381*, which mediates tetracycline and minocycline resistance via the *tetM* gene (Rice *et al.*, 1992). Such elements are prevalent in streptococci as well as enterococci, and have been shown to possess an extremely broad host range that has likely contributed to the wide distribution of *tetM* alleles among both Gram-positive and Gram-negative bacterial genera (Salyers and Amábile-Cuevas, 1997; Rice, 1998).

To the right of the internal IS*1216* copy is a DNA segment with similarity to a relaxase gene of mobilisable plasmids from staphylococci (Bonafede *et al.*, 1997). This plasmid remnant is flanked by a copy of the aminoglycoside resistance transposon Tn*4001* (see above)(Rice *et al.*, 1995). Adjacent to and truncated by the leftmost copy of IS*256* in Tn*4001* are sequences identical to the replication region of the broad-host range plasmid pAMβ1 (Bonafede *et al.*, 1997). This plasmid remnant is also bisected by a Tn*917*-like transposon that confers resistance to MLS antibiotics via an *ermAM* determinant (Bonafede *et al.*, 1997).

The right-hand end of Tn*5385*, bounded by the third copy of IS*1216*, possesses sequences and an organization typical of staphylococcal β-lactamase/heavy-metal resistance plasmids (Rice *et al.*, 1996; Bonafede *et al.*, 1997; Firth and Skurray, 2000). Namely, an IS*257*-flanked segment encoding a *merA-merB* operon which confers resistance to mercury/organomercurials (see above) and a Tn*552*-like β-lactamase transposon adjacent to a resolvase gene (Rice *et al.*, 1996; Bonafede *et al.*, 1997); Tn*552* belongs to a group of transposons that appear to insert preferentially at resolution sites (Paulsen *et al.*, 1994; Berg *et al.*, 1998; Minakhina *et al.*, 1999). The third copy of IS*256* within Tn*5385* is located within this Tn*552*-like element, inserted into *blaR1*, a sensor protein involved in the regulation of the divergently transcribed upstream *blaZ* β-lactamase gene (Rice and Marshall, 1994; Rice *et al.*, 1996). The internal segment of Tn*5385* bounded by this copy of IS*256* at one end, and the leftmost copy of IS*256* from Tn*4001* at the other, forms a composite structure designated Tn*5384*, which has been shown to transpose as a unit (Rice *et al.*, 1995).

Tn*5385* is clearly the product of a complex evolutionary pathway (Rice, 2000). It is likely, however, that this pathway has involved a series of cointegration events between plasmids, of potentially diverse origins, mediated by transposable elements, particularly IS*1216*. Other events mediated by transposable elements have further shaped the structure of Tn*5385*. Insertion sequence-mediated deletion events appear to be responsible for the removal of segments of redundant and/or potentially metabolically burdensome plasmid DNA, including several plasmid replication and transfer regions. Additionally, the insertion of IS*256* into the β-lactamase regulatory gene and the insertions of the Tn*917*-like transposon and possibly Tn*4001* into plasmid replication functions likely represent cases of insertional inactivation. In such instances, it is likely that it is the inactivation that confers the initial evolutionary advantage rather than any antimicrobial resistance gene carried by the transposon, which is presumably exploited to advantage subsequently.

The series of events described above has resulted not only in assembly of Tn*5385*, but also in the generation of Tn*5384* which is capable of moving the aminoglycoside, MLS and mercury resistance determinants that it contains as part of a bona fide composite transposon (Rice *et al.*, 1995). Formal transposition of Tn*5385* has not yet been demonstrated. Rather, insertion into a target DNA molecule has been observed via homologous recombination involving flanking sequences or copies of Tn*5381* present within Tn*5385* and the target DNA (Rice and Carias, 1998). The mechanism by which Tn*5385* is able to move intercellularly is also not understood, but may rely on conjugative functions provided by the internal copy of Tn*5381* (Rice and Carias, 1998).

When considering the significance of structures like Tn*5385*, it should be recognised that the element that has been characterised may represent a terminal "dead end" branch of an ongoing evolutionary pathway. So, for example, although Tn*5385* was found chromosomally and lacks a broad-host range conjugation and replication system normally associated with pAMβ1-like plasmids, these functions may only have been discarded in the clinical strain that was identified and subsequently studied. The broad-host range conjugative plasmid from which Tn*5385* likely descended may well still exist and continue to be playing a role in the dissemination of multi-resistance. Similarly, since detailed studies of elements such as Tn*5385* are usually based on very limited numbers of strains, representing only one of a range of cohabiting potential host species or genera, it is likely that we are only glimpsing isolated snapshots of a spectrum of existing multi-resistance structures.

The Role of Selection

The examples described above illustrate the capacity of mobile genetic elements to mediate the recruitment of antimicrobial resistance genes and assemble them into multi-resistance clusters. Although mobile elements have clearly been fundamental to the evolution of multi-resistance in many genera, their role is essentially one of passive facilitation. They are merely tools to generate sufficient genetic variation upon which selection ultimately arbitrates. The prevalence of multi-resistance structures does not reflect the efficiency of their production, but rather demonstrates the power of prevailing selection to amplify the single cell that carries such a structure by preventing the growth of all other cells that don't. The assembly or resistance gene clusters is a demonstration of selection operating not only at the level of organisms, but simultaneously at the level of genes and DNA molecules (Eberhard, 1990). Resistance genes become associated with each other because in an environment of varying antimicrobial selection it is evolutionarily advantageous to the genes themselves to be horizontally transmissible as a genetically linked unit, since it maximizes the likelihood of their establishment in new hosts. An equivalent advantage is conferred on a plasmid which carries multiple resistance genes.

Multi-resistant strains that now plague mankind have not become such a problem because they have tools that allow them to become multi-resistant, they have become so prevalent because mankind has so effectively created conditions that preferentially select for their survival. Although the relationship between the use of antimicrobial agents and the emergence of resistance was described soon after the therapeutic introduction of antibiotics, the use of these agents globally can still at best be described as a haphazard. Widespread recognition of the fundamental role of selection in the development of resistance, underpinned by an appreciation of the capacity of microbes to adapt to environmental challenges, is essential if we are to maximize the effectiveness of precious current and future antimicrobial resources.

Acknowledgements

Work in the Laboratory of N.F. was supported by Project Grant 153816 from the National Health and Medical Research Council (Australia).

References

Allignet, J. and El Solh, N. 1999. Comparative analysis of staphylococcal plasmids carrying three streptogramin-resistance genes: *vat-vgb-vga*. Plasmid. 42: 134-138.

Apisiridej, S., Leelaporn, A., Scaramuzzi, C.D., Skurray, R.A. and Firth, N. 1997. Molecular analysis of a mobilizable theta-mode trimethoprim resistance plasmid from coagulase-negative staphylococci. Plasmid. 38: 13-24.

Archer, G.L. and Niemeyer, D.M. 1994. Origin and evolution of DNA associated with resistance to methicillin in staphylococci. Trends Microbiol. 2: 343-347.

Archer, G.L. and Thomas Jr., W.D. 1990. Conjugative transfer of antimicrobial resistance genes between staphylococci. In: Molecular Biology of the Staphylococci. R.P. Novick, ed. VCH, New York. p. 115-122.

Bannam, T.L. and Rood, J.I. 1991. Relationship between the *Clostridium perfringens catQ* gene product and chloramphenicol acetyltransferases from other bacteria. Antimicrob. Agents Chemother. 35: 471-476.

Berg, T., Firth, N., Apisiridej, S., Hettiaratchi, A., Leelaporn, A. and Skurray, R.A. 1998. Complete nucleotide sequence of pSK41: evolution of staphylococcal conjugative plasmids. J. Bacteriol. 180: 4350-4359.

Bonafede, M.E., Carias, L.L. and Rice, L.B. 1997. Enterococcal transposon Tn*5384* - evolution of a composite transposon through cointegration of enterococcal and staphylococcal plasmids. Antimicrob. Agents Chemother. 41: 1854-1858.

Byrne, M.E., Gillespie, M.T. and Skurray, R.A. 1990. Molecular analysis of a gentamicin resistance transposonlike element on plasmids isolated from North American *Staphylococcus aureus* strains. Antimicrob. Agents Chemother. 34: 2106-2113.

Byrne, M.E., Gillespie, M.T. and Skurray, R.A. 1991. 4',4'' adenyltransferase activity on conjugative plasmids isolated from *Staphylococcus aureus* is encoded on an integrated copy of pUB110. Plasmid. 25: 70-75.

Cetinkaya, Y., Falk, P. and Mayhall, C.G. 2000. Vancomycin-resistant enterococci. Clin. Microbiol. Rev. 13: 686-707.

Chopra, I. 1976. Mechanisms of resistance to fusidic acid in *Staphylococcus aureus*. J. Gen. Microbiol. 96: 229-238.

Clermont, D., Chesneau, O., de Cespédès, G. and Horaud, T. 1997. New tetracycline resistance determinants coding for ribosomal protection in streptococci and nucleotide sequence of *tet*(T) isolated from *Streptococcus pyogenes* A498. Antimicrob. Agents Chemother. 41: 112-116.

Crupper, S.S., Worrell, V., Stewart, G.C. and Iandolo, J.J. 1999. Cloning and expression of *cadD*, a new cadmium resistance gene of *Staphylococcus aureus*. J. Bacteriol. 181: 4071-4075.

Day, N.P., Moore, C.E., Enright, M.C., Berendt, A.R., Smith, J.M., Murphy, M.F., Peacock, S.J., Spratt, B.G. and Feil, E.J. 2001. A link between virulence and ecological abundance in natural populations of *Staphylococcus aureus*. Science. 292: 114-116.

Dubin, D.T., Chikramane, S.G., Inglis, B., Matthews, P.R. and Stewart, P.R. 1992. Physical mapping of the *mec* region of an Australian methicillin-resistant *Staphylococcus aureus* lineage and a closely related American strain. J. Gen. Microbiol. 138: 169-180.

Dyke, K.G., Aubert, S. and El Solh, N. 1992. Multiple copies of IS*256* in staphylococci. Plasmid. 28: 235-246.

Eberhard, W.G. 1990. Evolution in bacterial plasmids and levels of selection. Quart. Rev. Biol. 65: 3-22.

Evans, J. and Dyke, K.G. 1988. Characterization of the conjugation system associated with the *Staphylococcus aureus* plasmid pJE1. J. Gen. Microbiol. 134: 1-8.

Feil, E.J., Holmes, E.C., Bessen, D.E., Chan, M.S., Day, N.P., Enright, M.C., Goldstein, R., Hood, D.W., Kalia, A., Moore, C.E., Zhou, J. and Spratt, B.G. 2001. Recombination within natural populations of pathogenic bacteria: short-term empirical estimates and long-term phylogenetic consequences. Proc. Natl. Acad. Sci. USA. 98: 182-187.

Firth, N., Apisiridej, S., Berg, T., O'Rourke, B.A., Curnock, S., Dyke, K.G.H. and Skurray, R.A. 2000. Replication of staphylococcal multiresistance plasmids. J. Bacteriol. 182: 2170-2178.

Firth, N. and Skurray, R.A. 1998. Mobile elements in the evolution and spread of multiple-drug resistance in staphylococci. Drug Resist. Updates. 1: 49-58.

Firth, N. and Skurray, R.A.. 2000. The *Staphylococcus* - genetics: accessory elements and genetic exchange. In: Gram-Positive Pathogens. V.A. Fischetti, R.P. Novick, J. Ferretti, D. Portnoy and J.I. Rood, eds. American Society for Microbiology, Washington, D.C. p. 326-338.

Fitzgerald, J.R., Sturdevant, D.E., Mackie, S.M., Gill, S.R. and Musser, J.M. 2001. Evolutionary genomics of *Staphylococcus aureus*: insights into the origin of methicillin-resistant strains and the toxic shock syndrome epidemic. Proc. Natl. Acad. Sci. USA. 98: 8821-8826.

Fontana, R., Aldegheri, M., Ligozzi, M., Lopez, H., Sucari, A. and Satta, G. 1994. Overproduction of a low-affinity penicillin-binding protein and high-level ampicillin resistance in *Enterococcus faecium*. Antimicrob. Agents Chemother. 38: 1980-1983.

Forbes, B.A. and Schaberg, D.R. 1983. Transfer of resistance plasmids from *Staphylococcus epidermidis* to *Staphylococcus aureus*: evidence for conjugative exchange of resistance. J. Bacteriol. 153: 627-634.

Gering, M., Götz, F. and Bruckner, R. 1996. Sequence and analysis of the replication region of the *Staphylococcus xylosus* plasmid pSX267. Gene 182: 117-122.

Gillespie, M.T., Lyon, B.R., Loo, L.S.L., Matthews, P.R., Stewart, P.R. and Skurray, R.A. 1987. Homologous direct repeat sequences associated with mercury, methicillin, tetracycline and trimethoprim resistance determinants in *Staphylococcus aureus*. FEMS Microbiol. Lett. 43: 165-171.

Gillespie, M.T., May, J.W. and Skurray, R.A. 1986. Detection of an integrated tetracycline resistance plasmid in the chromosome of methicillin-resistant *Staphylococcus aureus*. J. Gen. Microbiol. 132: 1723-1728.

Hartman, B.J. and Tomasz, A. 1984. Low-affinity penicillin-binding protein associated with β-lactam resistance in *Staphylococcus aureus*. J. Bacteriol. 158: 513-516.

Helinski, D.R., Toukdarian, A.E. and Novick, R.P. 1996. Replication control and other stable maintenance mechanisms of plasmids. In: *Escherichia coli* and *Salmonella*: Cellular and Molecular Biology. F.C. Neidhardt, R. Curtiss, J.L. Ingraham, E.C.C. Lin, K.B. Low, Jr., B. Magasanik, W. Reznikoff, M. Riley, M. Schaechter and H.E. Umbarger, eds. American Society for Microbiology, Washington, D.C., p. 2295-2324.

Hiramatsu, K., Cui, L., Kuroda, M. and Ito, T. 2001. The emergence and evolution of methicillin-resistant *Staphylococcus aureus*. Trends Microbiol. 9: 486-493.

Hodel-Christian, S.L. and Murray, B.E. 1991. Characterization of the gentamicin resistance transposon Tn*5281* from *Enterococcus faecalis* and comparison to staphylococcal transposons Tn*4001* and Tn*4031*. Antimicrob. Agents Chemother. 35: 1147-1152.

Horaud, T., de Cespédès, G. and Trieu-Cuot, P. 1996. Chromosomal gentamicin resistance transposon Tn*3706* in *Streptococcus agalactiae* B128. Antimicrob. Agents Chemother. 40: 1085-1090.

Ito, T., Katayama, Y., Asada, K., Mori, N., Tsutsumimoto, K., Tiensasitorn, C. and Hiramatsu, K. 2001. Structural comparison of three types of staphylococcal cassette chromosome *mec* integrated in the chromosome in methicillin-resistant *Staphylococcus aureus*. Antimicrob. Agents Chemother. 45: 1323-1336.

Ito, T., Katayama, Y. and Hiramatsu, K. 1999. Cloning and nucleotide sequence determination of the entire *mec* DNA of pre-methicillin-resistant *Staphylococcus aureus* N315. Antimicrob. Agents Chemother. 43: 1449-1458.

Jarlier, V. and Nikaido, H. 1994. Mycobacterial cell wall: structure and role in natural resistance to antibiotics. FEMS Microbiol, Lett. 123: 11-18.

Katayama, Y., Ito, T. and Hiramatsu, K. 2000. A new class of genetic element, staphylococcus cassette chromosome *mec*, encodes methicillin resistance in *Staphylococcus aureus*. Antimicrob. Agents Chemother.44: 1549-1555.

Katayama, Y., Ito, T. and Hiramatsu, K. 2001. Genetic organization of the chromosome region surrounding *mecA* in clinical staphylococcal strains: role of IS*431*-mediated *mecI* deletion in expression of resistance in *mecA*-carrying, low-level methicillin-resistant *Staphylococcus haemolyticus*. Antimicrob. Agents Chemother. 45: 1955-1963.

Kobayashi, N., Taniguchi, K. and Urasawa, S. 1998. Analysis of diversity of mutations in the *mecI* gene and *mecA* promoter/operator region of methicillin-resistant *Staphylococcus aureus* and *Staphylococcus epidermidis*. Antimicrob. Agents Chemother. 42: 717-720.

Kobayashi, N., Urasawa, S., Uehara, N. and Watanabe, N. 1999. Distribution of insertion sequence-like element IS*1272* and its position relative to methicillin resistance genes in clinically important staphylococci. Antimicrob. Agents Chemother. 43: 2780-2782.

Lacey, R.W. 1980. Evidence for two mechanisms of plasmid transfer in mixed cultures of *Staphylococcus aureus*. J. Gen. Microbiol. 119: 423-435.

Laddaga, R.A., Chu, L., Misra, T.K. and Silver, S. 1987. Nucleotide sequence and expression of the mercurial-resistance operon from *Staphylococcus aureus* plasmid pI258. Proc. Natl. Acad. Sci. USA. 84: 5106-5110.

Leelaporn, A., Firth, N., Byrne, M.E., Roper, E. and Skurray, R.A.. 1994. Possible role of insertion sequence IS*257* in dissemination and expression of high- and low-level trimethoprim resistance in staphylococci. Antimicrob. Agents Chemother. 38: 2238-2244.

Leelaporn, A., Firth, N., Paulsen, I.T. and Skurray, R.A. 1996. IS*257*-mediated cointegration in the evolution of a family of staphylococcal trimethoprim resistance plasmids. J. Bacteriol. 178: 6070-6073.

Littlejohn, T.G., DiBerardino, D., Messerotti, L.J., Spiers, S.J. and Skurray, R.A. 1991. Structure and evolution of a family of genes encoding antiseptic and disinfectant resistance in *Staphylococcus aureus*. Gene 101: 59-66.

Lyon, B.R., Gillespie, M.T. and Skurray, R.A. 1987. Detection and characterization of IS*256*, an insertion sequence in *Staphylococcus aureus*. J. Gen. Microbiol. 133: 3031-3038.

Lyon, B.R. and Skurray, R. 1987. Antimicrobial resistance of *Staphylococcus aureus*: genetic basis. Microbiol. Rev. 51: 88-134.

Macrina, F.L. and Archer, G.L. 1993. Conjugation and broad host range plasmids in streptococci and staphylococci. In: Bacterial Conjugation. D.B. Clewell, ed. Plenum Press, New York, USA. p. 313-329.

Mahillon, J. and Chandler, M. 1998. Insertion sequences. Microbiol. Mol. Biol. Rev. 62: 725-774.

McDonnell, R.W., Sweeney, H.M. and Cohen, S. 1983. Conjugational transfer of gentamicin resistance plasmids intra- and interspecifically in *Staphylococcus aureus* and *Staphylococcus epidermidis*. Antimicrob. Agents Chemother. 23: 151-160.

Minakhina, S., Kholodii, G., Mindlin, S., Yurieva, O. and Nikiforov, V. 1999. Tn*5053* family transposons are *res* site hunters sensing plasmidal *res* sites occupied by cognate resolvases. Mol. Microbiol. 33: 1059-1068.

Morton, T.M., Eaton, D.M., Johnston, J.L. and Archer, G.L. 1993. DNA sequence and units of transcription of the conjugative transfer gene complex (*trs*) of *Staphylococcus aureus* plasmid pGO1. J. Bacteriol. 175: 4436-4447.

Morton, T.M., Johnston, J.L., Patterson, J. and Archer, G.L. 1995. Characterization of a conjugative staphylococcal mupirocin resistance plasmid. Antimicrob. Agents Chemother. 39: 1272-1280.

Murphy, E. 1985a. Nucleotide sequence of a spectinomycin adenyltransferase AAD(9) determinant from *Staphylococcus aureus* and its relationship to AAD(3") (9). Mol. Gen. Genet. 200: 33-39.

Murphy, E. 1985b. Nucleotide sequence of *ermA*, a macrolide-lincosamide-streptogramin B determinant in *Staphylococcus aureus*. J. Bacteriol. 162: 633-640.

Needham, C., Noble, W.C. and Dyke, K.G.H. 1995. The staphylococcal insertion sequence IS*257* is active. Plasmid. 34: 198-205.

Needham, C., Rahman, M., Dyke, K.G.H. and Noble, W.C. 1994. An investigation of plasmids from *Staphylococcus aureus* that mediate resistance to mupirocin and tetracycline. Microbiol. 140: 2577-2583.

Nesvera, J., Hochmannova, J. and Patek, M. 1998. An integron of class 1 is present on the plasmid pCG4 from gram-positive bacterium *Corynebacterium glutamicum*. FEMS Microbiol. Lett. 169: 391-395.

Niemeyer, D.M., Pucci, M.J., Thanassi, J.A., Sharma, V.K. and Archer, G.L. 1996. Role of *mecA* transcriptional regulation in the phenotypic expression of methicillin resistance in *Staphylococcus aureus*. J. Bacteriol. 178: 5464-5471.

Novick, R.P. 1989. Staphylococcal plasmids and their replication. Ann. Rev. Microbiol. 43: 537-565.

Ochman, H., Lawrence, J.G. and Groisman, E.A. 2000. Lateral gene transfer and the nature of bacterial innovation. Nature. 405: 299-304.

Oliveira, D.C., Wu, S.W. and de Lencastre, H. 2000. Genetic organization of the downstream region of the *mecA* element in methicillin-resistant *Staphylococcus aureus* isolates carrying different polymorphisms of this region. Antimicrob. Agents Chemother. 44: 1906-1910.

Paulsen, I.T., Firth, N. and Skurray, R.A. 1997. Resistance to antimicrobial agents other than β-lactams. In: The Staphylococci in Human Disease. K.B. Crossley and G.L. Archer, eds. Churchill Livingstone, New York. p. 175-212.

Paulsen, I.T., Gillespie, M.T., Littlejohn, T.G., Hanvivatvong, O., Rowland, S.J., Dyke, K.G. and Skurray, R.A. 1994. Characterisation of *sin*, a potential recombinase-encoding gene from *Staphylococcus aureus*. Gene 141: 109-114.

Projan, S.J. and Archer, G.L. 1989. Mobilization of the relaxable *Staphylococcus aureus* plasmid pC221 by the conjugative plasmid pGO1 involves three pC221 loci. J. Bacteriol. 171: 1841-1845.

Rice, L.B. 1998. Tn*916* family conjugative transposons and dissemination of antimicrobial resistance determinants. Antimicrob. Agents Chemother. 42: 1871-1877.

Rice, L.B. 2000. Bacterial monopolists: the bundling and dissemination of antimicrobial resistance genes in gram-positive bacteria. Clin. Infect. Dis. 31: 762-769.

Rice, L.B. and Carias, L.L. 1998. Transfer of Tn*5385*, a composite, multiresistance chromosomal element from *Enterococcus faecalis*. J. Bacteriol. 180: 714-21.

Rice, L.B., Carias, L.L. and Marshall, S.H. 1995. Tn*5384*, a composite enterococcal mobile element conferring resistance to erythromycin and gentamicin whose ends are directly repeated copies of IS*256*. Antimicrob. Agents Chemother. 39: 1147-1153.

Rice, L.B., Carias, L.L., Marshall, S.H. and Bonafede, M.E. 1996. Sequences found on staphylococcal β-lactamase plasmids integrated into the chromosome of *Enterococcus faecalis* CH116. Plasmid 35: 81-90.

Rice, L.B. and Marshall, S.H. 1994. Insertions of IS*256*-like element flanking the chromosomal β–lactamase gene of *Enterococcus-faecalis* CX19. Antimicrob. Agents Chemother. 38: 693-701.

Rice, L.B., Marshall, S.H. and Carias, L.L. 1992. Tn*5381*, a conjugative transposon identifiable as a circular form in *Enterococcus faecalis*. J. Bacteriol. 174: 7308-7315.

Rice, L.B. and Thorisdottir, A.S. 1994. Prevalence of sequences homologous to IS256 in clinical enterococcal isolates. Plasmid 32: 344-349.

Rouch, D.A., Byrne, M.E., Kong, Y.C. and Skurray, R.A. 1987. The aacA-aphD gentamicin and kanamycin resistance determinant of Tn4001 from Staphylococcus aureus: expression and nucleotide sequence analysis. J. Gen. Microbiol. 133: 3039-3052.

Rouch, D.A., Messerotti, L.J., Loo, L.S., Jackson, C.A. and Skurray, R.A. 1989. Trimethoprim resistance transposon Tn4003 from Staphylococcus aureus encodes genes for a dihydrofolate reductase and thymidylate synthetase flanked by three copies of IS257. Mol. Microbiol. 3: 161-175.

Sadaie, Y., Burtis, K.C. and Doi, R.H. 1980. Purification and characterization of a kanamycin nucleotidyltransferase from plasmid pUB110-carrying cells of Bacillus subtilis. J. Bacteriol. 141: 1178-1182.

Salyers, A.A. and Amábile-Cuevas, C.F. 1997. Why are antibiotic resistance genes so resistant to elimination? Antimicrob. Agents Chemother. 41: 2321-2325.

Semon, D., Movva, M.R. and Smith, T.F. 1987. Plasmid-determined bleomycin resistance in Staphylococcus aureus. Plasmid 17: 46-53.

Sharma, V.K., Hackbarth, C.J., Dickinson, T.M. and Archer, G.L. 1998. Interaction of native and mutant MecI repressors with sequences that regulate mecA, the gene encoding penicillin binding protein 2a in methicillin-resistant staphylococci. J. Bacteriol. 180: 2160-2166.

Simpson, A.E., Skurray, R.A. and Firth, N. 2000. An IS257-derived hybrid promoter directs transcription of a tetA(K) tetracycline resistance gene in the Staphylococcus aureus chromosomal mec region. J. Bacteriol. 182: 3345-3352.

Skurray, R.A. and Firth, N. 1997. Molecular evolution of multiply-antibiotic-resistant staphylococci. CIBA Found. Symp. 207: 167-183.

Somoskovi, A., Parsons, L.M. and Salfinger, M. 2001. The molecular basis of resistance to isoniazid, rifampin, and pyrazinamide in Mycobacterium tuberculosis. Respir. Res. 2: 164-168.

Song, M.D., Wachi, M., Doi, M., Ishino, F. and Matsuhashi, M. 1987. Evolution of an inducible penicillin-target protein in methicillin-resistant Staphylococcus aureus by gene fusion. FEBS Lett. 221: 167-171.

Stewart, P.R., Dubin, D.T., Chikramane, S.G., Inglis, B., Matthews, P.R. and Poston, S.M. 1994. IS*257* and small plasmid insertions in the *mec* region of the chromosome of *Staphylococcus aureus*. Plasmid 31: 12-20.

Sugiyama, M., Kumagai, T., Matsuo, H., Bhuiyan, M.Z., Ueda, K., Mochizuki, H., Nakamura, N. and Davies, J.E. 1995. Overproduction of the bleomycin-binding proteins from bleomycin- producing *Streptomyces verticillus* and a methicillin-resistant *Staphylococcus aureus* in *Escherichia coli* and their immunological characterisation. FEBS Lett. 362: 80-84.

Thomas Jr., W.D. and Archer, G.L. 1992. Mobilization of recombinant plasmids from *Staphylococcus aureus* into coagulase negative *Staphylococcus* species. Plasmid 27: 164-168.

Werckenthin, C., Schwarz, S. and Roberts, M.C. 1996. Integration of pT181-like tetracycline resistance plasmids into large staphylococcal plasmids involves IS*257*. Antimicrob. Agents Chemother. 40: 2542-2544.

Witte, W., Green, L., Misra, T.K. and Silver, S. 1986. Resistance to mercury and to cadmium in chromosomally resistant *Staphylococcus aureus*. Antimicrob. Agents Chemother. 29: 663-669.

Wu, S., de Lencastre, H. and Tomasz, A. 1998. Genetic organization of the *mecA* region in methicillin-susceptible and methicillin-resistant strains of *Staphylococcus sciuri*. J. Bacteriol. 180: 236-242.

Wu, S., Piscitelli, C., de Lencastre, H. and Tomasz, A. 1996. Tracking the evolutionary origin of the methicillin resistance gene: cloning and sequencing of a homologue of *mecA* from a methicillin susceptible strain of *Staphylococcus sciuri*. Microbial Drug Resist. 2: 435-441.

Yamaguchi, A., Shiina, Y., Fujihira, E., Sawai, T., Noguchi, N. and Sasatsu, M. 1995. The tetracycline efflux protein encoded by the *tet*(K) gene from *Staphylococcus aureus* is a metal-tetracycline/H$^+$ antiporter. FEBS Lett. 365: 193-197.

Young, H.K., Skurray, R.A. and Amyes, S.G. 1987. Plasmid-mediated trimethoprim-resistance in *Staphylococcus aureus*. Characterization of the first gram-positive plasmid dihydrofolate reductase (type S1). Biochem. J. 243: 309-312.

Zhang, Y. and Young, D. 1994. Molecular genetics of drug resistance in *Mycobacterium tuberculosis*. J. Antimicrob. Chemother. 34: 313-319.

From: *Multiple Drug Resistant Bacteria*
Edited by: Carlos F. Amábile-Cuevas

Chapter 4

Multiple Resistance Mediated by Individual Genetic Loci

Bruce Demple and
Carlos F. Amábile-Cuevas

Abstract

In addition to the clustering of single-drug-resistance genes, and to the decreased susceptibility to antibiotics displayed by biofilms, multi-resistance can arise as the consequence of the activation of stress responses, or mutations in regulatory genes governing those responses. Two regulons originally characterized in *E. coli* but known to be present in other gram-negative bacteria, confer multi-resistance when activated, usually by non-antibiotic agents: *marRAB* and *soxRS*. The resistance phenotype is caused by both, decreased permeability of the outer membrane, and by the expression of efflux pumps. Regulatory proteins of both systems share great homology, and the regulons overlap to some extent. Mutations affecting these regulatory genes, resulting in constitutive expression of the regulons, can also confer multi-resistance.

Such mutants have been isolated from antibiotic-resistant infections, although the epidemiological relevance of such organisms remains to be established. Other proteins, homologous to MarA or SoxS, when overexpressed, are capable of diminishing the susceptibility to antibiotics; plasmids bearing *mar*, *sox*, or homologous genes, are now only laboratory constructs, but could be naturally selected for by several environmental pressures, including but not limited to antibiotics.

Introduction

The previous chapters discussed how gene mobilization could result in the gathering of resistance determinants in a single genetic element or a single cell. This section is devoted to the description of single genes conferring multiple resistance. The first two examples are regulatory genes found in gram-negative bacteria. The responses they regulate confer multiple antibiotic resistance, and mutations resulting in the constitutive expression of such responses render the mutant bacteria permanently resistant. Furthermore, the transient switching-on of these systems can protect the bacterial cell against antimicrobial drugs; since agents capable of eliciting these responses are mainly non-antibiotic compounds, such agents may pose an unexpected selective pressure favoring antibiotic resistance.

Other single loci conferring multiple resistance include those affecting the permeability of the outer membrane of gram-negative organisms, and those encoding efflux pumps. In addition to physiological regulation of permeability and efflux mechanisms, they may be directly affected by mutations in their own genes to produce a multiple-antibiotic resistance phenotype. *Pseudomonas aeruginosa*, for instance, is a dangerous organism causing hospital-acquired infections, often resistant to most available antibiotics due to the over-expression of a variety of efflux pumps (Livermore, 2002).

Stress Responses Affecting Antibiotic Resistance: The *marRAB* and *soxRS* Regulons

As single-cell organisms, bacteria need to cope with environmental stress in a quick, efficient manner. Dramatic changes in environmental conditions are common in the life of a bacterium: for example, in minutes bacteria can go from the intestinal habitat (37°C, available nutrients, iso-osmolarity) to sewage (usually <20°C, noxious chemicals such as chlorine, detergents and disinfectants, variable concentrations of nutrients and salts). Physical or chemical signals that trigger the expression of defense mechanisms often have overlapping effects, so that response to a single stimulus may provide protection to a wide variety of environmental conditions. These stress responses include systems that protect the bacterial cell against heat, cold, osmolarity changes, starvation, oxidants, etc. In this section, two overlapping stress-defense systems that provide unspecific antibiotic resistance will be described: the *marRAB* regulon, responding to a number of xenobiotic agents; and the *soxRS* regulon, responding to superoxide stress. Although most studies on these regulated systems have been made with *Escherichia coli*, other gram-negative bacteria bear similar mechanisms. Furthermore, clinical isolates from patients with infections that have not yielded to antimicrobial therapy, contain bacterial pathogens with *sox-* or *mar*-constitutive mutations. However, the complete role of these mechanisms in furnishing bacteria with transient protection against antibiotics is yet to be established.

Multiple Antibiotic Resistance: MarRAB

A chromosomal multiple antibiotic resistance (Mar) system was described in 1983 by George and Levy in *E. coli*. Mutations could be selected by a single drug (*e.g.*, chloramphenicol or tetracycline), but conferred resistance to unrelated compounds, such as β-lactams or nalidixic acid. Transposon-mutagenesis identified the locus, named *marA*, at 34 min on the *E. coli* chromosome map (George and Levy, 1983a, 1983b). Independently isolated mutations conferring Mar were located at the same chromosomal locus: a mutation conferring some of the phenotypes associated with *soxRS*-mutants (see below), called *soxQ* (Greenberg *et al.*, 1991); and *cfxB*, conferring resistance to quinolones resulting from reduced drug accumulation (Hooper *et al.*, 1989). Multi-resistance induced by salicylates (Rosner, 1985), was also found to be mediated by the *mar* locus.

The *mar* locus (Figure 1) consists of two divergently transcribed units, *marC* and *marRAB*. Independent promoters (Pmar$_I$ for *marC*, and Pmar$_{II}$ for *marRAB*) are located in the *marC-marR* intergenic region. The function of the MarC protein is unknown; its deduced amino acid sequence suggests that the protein may be located inside the

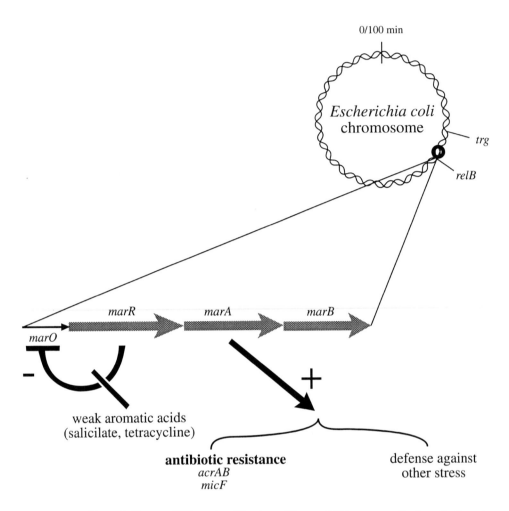

Figure 1. The *marRAB* regulon. Structure of the *marRAB* operon, activating stimili, and relevant known activated genes. Modified from Amábile-Cuevas and Fuentes (1996) by Isabel Nivón.

membrane. MarB is also a protein of unknown function (Barbosa and Levy, 2000). MarR acts as a repressor for the whole operon, and is likely to be the sensor for chemical stimuli. MarA is a positive regulator, the induction of which by de-repression results in the activation of the *mar* regulon genes (overlapped with the *soxRS* regulon) (Ariza et al., 1994). The *soxQ1*, *marR1* and *cfxB1* mutations are all located within the *marR* gene and yield a partial or total inactivation of MarR function (Ariza et al., 1994).

The activation of the *mar* regulon results in increased antibiotic resistance, along with resistance to organic solvents, disinfectants and oxidants. The Mar phenotype is caused both because of a decrease in the permeability of the outer membrane, and due to active efflux systems (McMurry *et al.*, 1994). The gene *micF* is positively regulated by MarA, and encodes an antisense RNA that binds to the *ompF* mRNA, which post-transcriptionally down-regulates expression of the OmpF porin. Inactivation of the *ompF* gene is sufficient by itself to produce a weak antibiotic resistance phenotype (Harder *et al.*, 1981). *micF* RNA levels increase in response to other stimuli, such as high temperature, high osmolarity and ethanol (Andersen *et al.*, 1989). On the other hand, the *acrAB* operon, which expression is activated by MarA, encodes for a complex efflux system that has been known to be involved in multi-resistance (Ma *et al.*, 1995). *acrB* encodes a multidrug transporter protein of the resistance-nodulation-cell division (RND) family, while AcrA is an associated protein of the membrane fusion protein (MFP) family (Putman *et al.*, 2000). Along with TolC, that seem to assemble into a "tunnel" that spans the outer membrane and periplasmic space, this extrusion system provides diminished susceptibility to several antibiotics including tetracycline, ampicillin (and other beta-lactams), chloramphenicol, rifampin, and fluoroquinolones (Webber and Piddock, 2001).

The *mar* locus regulates a step-by-step defense system against chemical insults; in addition to controlling *micF* and *acrAB* associated with antibiotic resistance, *mar* also regulates some of the *sox* regulon genes (see below). Actually, two independent experiments using microarray technology, showed that in addition to activating the genes noted above, MarA was found to be capable of increasing the expression of 47 genes, while the expression of another 15 was decreased (Barbosa and Levy, 2000); and salicylate treatment, known to specifically activate the *marRAB* regulon, increase the expression of 84 genes, and decrease the expression of 60 (Pomposiello *et al.*, 2001). These microarray experiments show that a wide variety of genes is affected by MarA overexpression; the biological significance of many of these genes being either repressed or activated under conditions that naturally affect MarR is still to be understood.

The recent evidence provided by microarray experiments clearly set apart the *mar* and *sox* regulons, previously considered to overlap extensively. However, the physiological overlap of *sox* and *mar* in terms of resistance phenotypes, still holds: antibiotics elicit both multiple antibiotic- and superoxide resistance, and superoxide-generating agents elicit both superoxide- and antibiotic resistance. Although part of this overlap may be attributed to the generation of oxygen radicals by some of the activating antibiotics (*e.g.*, tetracycline generates superoxide, hydrogen peroxide and hydroxyl radicals after its exposure to visible light, being these reactive species responsible for the phototoxicity of this antibiotic toward *E. coli* (Martin *et al.*, 1987)), this does not seems to hold for the majority of *mar* activators. But studies using experimental drugs apparently incapable of generating free radicals, selected a *soxR* mutant displaying antibiotic resistance, which partially depended on the presence of *mar* genes (Miller *et al.*, 1994). Work with *inaA*, a gene that is expressed after treating *E. coli* cells with weak acids, and that is governed both by *mar* and *sox*, support an interaction between the effector proteins of both regulons, MarA and SoxS: the levels of *inaA* induced by paraquat (a superoxide-generating agent) are 30-50% less in *mar* strains than in *mar*[+] strains (*soxRS* deletion, but not *mar* deletion, prevented the inducibility of *inaA* by paraquat) (Rosner and Slonczewski, 1994). Altogether, evidences point at intricate interactions, both at the physiological and genetic levels, between the *sox* and *mar* systems.

Superoxide Stress, SoxRS and Antibiotic Resistance

While characterizing a set of *E. coli* mutants that were resistant to menadione, a regulatory locus was detected: *soxR* (Greenberg *et al.*, 1990). Menadione-resistant mutants were those constitutively expressing the proteins encoded by the *soxR* regulon genes; therefore, it seems that this regulon plays a key role in the cellular defense against superoxide. The *soxRS* regulon is yet a component of a larger set of genes induced by superoxide, known as the superoxide stimulon. Under normal growth conditions, intracellular $O_2^{\cdot-}$ in *E. coli* is estimated to be limited to 2×10^{-10} M (Liochev and Fridovich, 1992b), *i.e.*, one or less molecules per cell. Most of these superoxide molecules come from natural or chemically induced "leaks" from the respiratory chain, and autoxidation of other cellular molecules. Additionally, bacterial cells are exposed to extracellular $O_2^{\cdot-}$ generated by activated macrophages during the "respiratory burst" (in addition to nitric oxide, $NO^{\cdot}$). The obvious and, perhaps, the first biochemical barrier against superoxide is superoxide-dismutase (SOD) activity. *E. coli* bears three different SODs: a constitutive, Fe-containing SOD, encoded by *sodB* (Fee, 1991); a more recently described CuZn-containing SOD, located in the periplasmic space, and expressed only during stationary phase, encoded by *sodC* (Benov and Fridovich, 1996, Imlay and Imlay, 1996); and an inducible, Mn-containing SOD. The *sodA* gene encoding Mn-SOD is part of the $O2^{\cdot-}$ stimulon (Fee, 1991). Fe-SOD and Mn-SOD catalyses the dismutation of intracellular superoxide, while CuZn-SOD inactivates $O2^{\cdot-}$ generated outside the cell. While Mn-SOD is synthesized during aerobiosis, Fe-SOD is formed even in the absence of oxygen; the proposed role of a SOD during anaerobiosis is to withstand a sudden change to aerobic conditions (Kargalioglu and Imlay, 1994). Components of anaerobic metabolism are known to generate superoxide when exposed to oxygen (a sort of "reperfusion damage"), so that the transition may represent a strong oxidative stress. Fe-SOD is more likely to be formed during anaerobiosis, due to the availability of iron (Kargalioglu and Imlay, 1994).

The *soxRS* regulon is also a multi-level defense system, mainly devoted to protect the cell against superoxide damage. Paraquat (PQ), a redox-cycling compound used experimentally to generate intracellular superoxide, induce the *soxRS* regulon; *E. coli* cells under PQ treatment, in microarray experiments, showed increased expression of 66 genes (while other 46 were down-regulated) (Pomposiello *et al.*, 2001). Genes clearly involved in superoxide defense include:

- *sodA*, encoding Mn-superoxide dismutase, and also induced by salicylate
- *nfo*, encoding endonuclease IV, a DNA-repair enzyme, not clearly shown in the microarray but known to be induced by PQ and governed by *soxRS* (Greenberg *et al.*, 1990)
- *zwf*, encoding glucose-6-P-dehydrogenase, possibly induced to replenish NADPH (Greenberg *et al.*, 1990)
- *fumC*, encoding a superoxide-resistant fumarase (Liochev and Fridovich, 1992a), also induced by salicylate
- *acnA*, encoding a superoxide-resistant aconitase (Gruer and Guest, 1994), also induced by salicylate.

Most interestingly, for the purposes of this chapter, both, *micF* and *acrAB*, mediating as previously discussed a multi-resistance phenotype, are also controlled by *soxRS*. *soxR*-constitutive mutants display a multi-resistance phenotype, and PQ and other superoxide-generating agents induce also such phenotype (Ariza *et al.*, 1994).

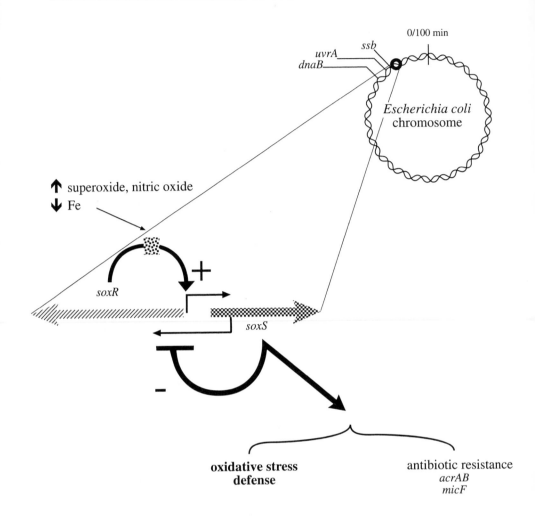

Figure 2. The *soxRS* regulon. Structure of the *soxRS* locus, activating stimuli, and relevant known activated genes. Modified from Amábile-Cuevas and Fuentes (1996) by Isabel Nivón.

The *soxRS* locus (Figure 2), located at minute 92 in *E. coli* chromosome, is composed by two divergently transcribed genes: *soxR* and *soxS*. The locus encompasses 874 bp with an 85-bp intergenic region containing promoters and regulatory elements. The *soxR* gene is a 465 bp sequence, encoding a 154-amino acid protein with a molecular weight of 17.1 kDa; the *soxS* gene is 324 bp in length, encoding a 107-amino acid, 12.9 kDa protein (Amábile-Cuevas and Demple, 1991). SoxR acts both as a sensor protein, and as a positive regulator of *soxS* expression, and represses its own gene, too (Hidalgo *et al.*, 1998); SoxS in turn activates the promoters of the *soxRS* regulon genes (Demple and Amábile-Cuevas, 1991) (and represses transcription of *soxS*) (Nunoshiba *et al.*, 1993b). This mini-cascade model of gene regulation was proposed based on the predicted homology between SoxR and SoxS and known gene regulators, and the ability of SoxS alone to activate several regulon genes in the absence of SoxR and superoxide stimulus, while SoxR alone was without effect (Amábile-Cuevas and Demple, 1991). As mentioned before, the two genes are divergently transcribed and the transcripts of the two genes overlap (Wu and Weiss, 1991). Experiments carried out with a *soxS'::lacZ* fusion supported the model of transcriptional regulation of *soxS* by activated SoxR protein: β-galactosidase activity increased in *soxR⁺,soxS'::lacZ* cells after treatment with paraquat, but no increase was detected in *soxR⁻* cells (Nunoshiba *et al.*, 1992). Increase in *soxS* mRNA content, after induction was also demonstrated (Wu and Weiss, 1991).

The amino acid sequence of SoxR protein shows homology with MerR (up to 29% identity in a 125-amino acid overlap). The homologous region includes a putative helix-turn-helix domain, as well a cluster of cysteine residues, that is responsible of mercury-binding in the MerR protein (Amábile-Cuevas and Demple, 1991). This cysteine cluster was proposed to be an iron-binding region in the SoxR protein, capable of sensing redox changes. In Fe-S proteins, iron ions may be bound to cysteine sulfur, or to inorganic S in a prosthetic group (iron-sulfur cluster). These Fe-S centers are often involved in electron transport, or in the catalytic activity of some enzymes (Roualt and Klausner, 1996). The actual existence of a Fe-S center was soon demonstrated (Hidalgo and Demple, 1994), and the nature of the reactions involved in the activation of SoxR ascertained. An apo-SoxR (devoid of Fe ions) is presumably turned into a dimer and then acquires a [2Fe-2S] center. The oxidation of the [2Fe-2S] centers activates SoxR (Ding *et al.*, 1997; Hidalgo and Demple, 1996a). Apo-SoxR and [2Fe-2S]-SoxR have the same affinity for the *soxS* promoter, and the presence of the metal is not necessary for RNA-polymerase binding, suggesting that the role of SoxR is to cause conformational changes in DNA, as proposed for MerR (Hidalgo *et al.*, 1995). In the presence of RNA-polymerase, activated SoxR causes a structural distortion of the promoter region, assisting RNA-polymerase in melting the DNA helix formed around position +1 (Hidalgo and Demple, 1996b).

Constitutive *soxRS* mutations have been isolated; these cells display high-level expression of the *soxRS*-regulon genes (or the *soxS'::lacZ* fusion). Mutations affect the C-terminus of the protein, but do not reach the cysteine-containing region (Nunoshiba and Demple, 1994). The indispensable role of cysteine residues in the SoxR protein has been demonstrated (Bradley et al., 1997). The mechanism by which the SoxR^c protein is kept active despite the oxidative state of the cell is unknown.

What is the nature of the SoxR activating signal? So far we know that intracellular superoxide-generating-agents (*i.e.*, aerobic paraquat) or conditions (augmented oxygen tension or diminished SOD), and extracellular nitric oxide (or related nitrous compounds, such as 4-nitroquinoline-*N*-oxide (Nunoshiba and Demple, 1993); see below) are capable of triggering the expression of *soxS*. Liochev *et al.* suggest that the ratio of reduced/oxidized "doxins" (*i.e.*, ferredoxins and flavodoxins) can be sensed by the iron-sulfur centers of SoxR, and may explain how many different agents and conditions are capable of SoxR-activation (Liochev *et al.*, 1994). A possible enzymatic step which may be responsible for the reduction (and, therefore the inactivation) of [2Fe-2S]-SoxR, requiring NADPH, has also been proposed (Hidalgo and Demple, 1994). A putative SoxR reductase has been reported (Kobayashi and Tagawa, 1999).

SoxR is also capable of sensing the intracellular levels of Fe^{2+}: when 2,2'-dipyridyl, an Fe^{2+}-chelating agent, is added, the SoxR-dependent expression of a *fumC'::lacZ* fusion is activated (Park and Gunsalus, 1995). Interestingly, the expression of a *soxS'::lacZ* fusion is not increased due to the chelating treatment; this result suggests that the Fe^{2+}-SoxR-mediated activation of the expression of *fumC* is not dependent on SoxS (Fuentes *et al.*, 2001). However, another iron chelator, 1,10-phenanthroline, did caused the anaerobic activation of *soxS* transcription (Privalle *et al.*, 1993). Iron metabolism and oxidative stress defenses act in a coordinate way (Zheng *et al.*, 1999).

Mercuric ions activate the expression of the *soxS'::lacZ* fusion, even in the absence of oxidative stress, or in cells carrying the SoxR^c protein (Fuentes and Amábile-Cuevas, 1997). Whether Hg^{2+} forms or stabilizes the SoxR dimer in a semi-active form, or simply increases the intracellular superoxide concentration remains to be established.

SoxS is a small protein -in fact, one of the smallest gene regulators known. It also contains a helix-turn-helix domain, likely to be responsible for its DNA-binding capabilities (Amábile-Cuevas and Demple, 1991), and its predicted amino acid sequence is homologous to other gene regulators. These proteins bind and activate several common proteins.

SoxS binds to the putative promoter regions of at least four *soxRS*-regulon genes, and recruits RNA polymerase to these regions (Li and Demple, 1994). SoxS also binds to the promoter region of its own gene, with a lower affinity, exerting a negative autoregulation (Nunoshiba *et al.*, 1993b). Gene activation by SoxS is "dose-dependent".

The overlapping region of homology between SoxS and AraC (and other members of this family of regulators) lies in their C-terminal region, while it covers almost the entire length of small proteins, such as MarA (discussed before) and TetD (related to tetracycline resistance, but of unknown function; see below). However, the homology with Rob protein, which binds to the right arm of the *E. coli* replication origin *oriC*, lies in the N-terminal region (Ariza *et al.*, 1995). Rob binds to several promoter regions of genes in the *soxRS* and *marRAB* regulons, although it does activate *in vitro* transcription of just some of them (Jair *et al.*, 1996b). Possible interactions between Rob, SoxS and MarA are being investigated: Why does Rob, present at 1000-5000 copies per cell under normal conditions, does not act upon *soxRS/marRAB* promoters *in vivo*? (Ariza *et al.*, 1995). The same authors suggest that the DNA-binding motif is an activator "module" used in different protein contexts (Ariza *et al.*, 1995), within a model of modular evolution of proteins.

In addition to the regulated genes shared by the *marRAB* and *soxRS* systems, the direct activator protein of both systems (MarA and SoxS, respectively) are very similar. MarA and SoxS, members of the AraC family of regulatory proteins, have strong amino acid sequence identity (up to 39%) (Gambino *et al.*, 1993), and similar DNA recognition and binding motifs, and transcriptional activation properties (Jair *et al.*, 1995). Both are also "ambidextrous" transcriptional activators, requiring the α C-terminal domain of RNA polymerase for activation of some of the genes they regulate (*zwf* and *fpr*) but not for *fumC* and *micF* (and *nfo* in the case of SoxS) (Jair *et al.*, 1995, 1996a).

Oxidative-stress response proteins have been proposed to be virulence mediators, since the reactive oxygen species they protect against are also released by activated macrophages (Hassett and Cohen, 1989). The *soxRS* regulon enhances the survival of *E. coli* within isolated macrophages, but the activating signal is nitric oxide rather than superoxide (Nunoshiba *et al.*, 1993a, 1995). A nitric oxide synthase is produced by macrophages upon activation. NO·, in turn, damages proteins and DNA, therefore being capable of severe cytotoxic effects. Interestingly enough, nitric oxide at much lower levels acts as an intercellular signaling molecule in mammalian systems. Extracellular NO˙ is capable of strongly inducing the expression of a *soxS'::lacZ* fusion, as well as several *soxRS*-regulated genes; in contrast, extracellular superoxide was unable to elicit these responses. The NO˙-dependent induction of *soxS'::lacZ* was even stronger under anaerobic conditions, eliminating the possible involvement of superoxide as an intermediate signal (Nunoshiba *et al.*, 1993a). Furthermore, *soxRS E. coli* cells were hypersensitive to the presence of activated murine macrophages, when compared to *soxRS⁺* cells (Nunoshiba *et al.*, 1993a). The exposure of cells bearing the *soxS'::lacZ* fusion to activated macrophages resulted in the induction of the gene fusion (Nunoshiba *et al.*, 1995). An *in vitro* model of NO˙ exposure that more closely mimics the output of activated macrophages (a continuous low-level flow, rather that a "bolus" exposure) resulted in higher expression of the *soxS'::lacZ* fusion (Nunoshiba *et al.*, 1995). Other possible level at which NO may be acting is changing the availability of iron ions: by changing Fe^{2+} into Fe^{3+}, macrophages diminish the iron uptake by bacteria (Sellers *et al.*, 1996). The lack of Fe^{2+} activates SoxR, as previously discussed, and it may also oxidize the Fe-S centers at SoxR dimers.

Inducible Resistance?

Clinical isolates displaying antibiotic resistance caused by mutations affecting the *marRAB* and —less frequently— the *soxRS* loci, have been described. These mutations result in the constitutive expression of the regulon genes. One of the first *marR* alleles was described from a ciprofloxacin-resistant *E. coli* clinical isolate, as previously discussed; and a *soxRS*-constitutive mutation was found to be responsible for antibiotic resistance in a *S. enterica* (serovar Typhimurium) clinical strain (Koutsolioutsou *et al.*, 2001). However, the contribution of *mar* and *sox* mutations to the overall resistance of clinically relevant bacteria has barely being explored. A rather small survey of fluoroquinolone-resistant *E. coli* showed that 10/36 overexpressed *soxS* and 5/36 overexpressed *marA*; but such changes did not seem to have a bearing upon the overexpression of the efflux system *acrAB*, supposedly responsible for the resistance phenotype (Webber and Piddock, 2001). But the overproduction of the AcrAB pump seems to appear earlier than *gyrA* mutations in yielding *S. enterica* serovar Typhimurium resistant to fluoroquinolones, although the possible role of *sox* or *mar* genes was not explored (Giraud *et al.*, 2000). Topoisomerase mutations alone, in the absence of the AcrAB efflux pump, did not confer clinically-relevant fluoroquinolone resistance in *E. coli* (Oethinger *et al.*, 2000). This field requires much more research to be done.

Moreover, the role of wild-type *marRAB* and *soxRS* genes in conferring inducible resistance of clinical relevance has not been confirmed. Hypothetical scenarios can easily be conceived: exposure to inducing stimuli (*e.g.*, environmental pollutants such as mercury, that activates the *soxRS* regulon; interactions between bacteria and macrophages, also affecting *sox* genes; decrease in iron availability, a known response to infectious processes, that again activates the *soxRS* regulon; non-antibiotic drugs such as aspirin, activating the *marRAB* regulon (Rosner, 1985)) shortly before antibiotic treatment, switches-on these defense mechanisms, protecting the bacterial cell against antibiotics. This protection might only be partial, but enough to allow bacteria to acquire other resistance determinants, by mutation or horizontal transfer; or acting along other protective conditions, such as growing in a biofilm (see next chapter). Experimental evidence of such effects might be obtained analyzing mRNA from bacteria causing actual infections.

A MarA-SoxS-like Protein Encoded by Mobile Genetic Elements

Amino acid sequence analyses showed that some other proteins of *E. coli* are quite similar to SoxS and MarA, as discussed before. One of them is TetD, a protein of yet unknown function (Pepe *et al.*, 1997). The *tetD* gene reside within the Tn*10* transposon, known to mediate tetracycline resistance (Braus *et al.*, 1984). Whether TetD activates *acrAB* or *micF* expression remains to be ascertained; but its homology to the amino acid sequence of SoxS is around 50%, and both proteins are of almost the same size (107 amino acids for SoxS, 103 for TetD) (Amábile-Cuevas and Demple, 1991). Tn*10* transposons bearing mutated *tetD* genes conferred similar tetracycline resistance than the wild-type transposon (Braus *et al.*, 1984); the same group reported TetD to be a membrane-associated protein, unlikely to exert a regulon-activating function. In any case, the possibility of such regulatory genes to "jump" to a mobilizable plasmid and confer a multi-resistance phenotype is disturbing.

Co-selection

Given that *marRAB* and *soxRS* are two systems devoted to cope with ancient kinds of environmental stress, it would seem likely that their primary function is (or was) not to confer antibiotic resistance. These regulatory genes seem to be conserved along a variety of gram-negative bacteria. The *mar* locus has been reported in *Salmonella*, *Shigella*, *Klebsiella*, *Citrobacter*, *Hafnia*, *Enterobacter* and, of course, in *E. coli* (Randall and Woodward, 2001). Both *soxR* and *soxS* were found only in *E. coli* and *S. enterica* serovar Typhimurium, but the chromosomes of *Pseudomonas aeruginosa* and *Vibrio cholerae* bear open reading frames encoding putative proteins homologous to SoxR (Fuentes *et al.*, 2001), and the complete sequences of very few organisms are available. Therefore, selective pressures other than the human use of antibiotics, selected and maintained these response mechanisms among a number of gamma-proteobacteria. Still, as the clinical relevance of inducible resistance remains to be ascertained, so is the role of pressures maintaining the wild-type regulatory mechanisms, upon the antibiotic resistance phenomenon. But non-antibiotic agents selecting for constitutive mutants of both regulons might be co-selecting for demonstrated clinically relevant antibiotic resistance. Disinfectant pine oil selects for *mar* mutants displaying a multi-resistance phenotype (Moken *et al.*, 1997). The overexpression of *marA* or *soxS* protects *E. coli* against another disinfectant, triclosan, now widely used in household materials (McMurry *et al.*, 1998). Ozone, at concentrations similar to those in polluted city air, might select for strains bearing *sox* genes, since   *soxRS* strains are more susceptible to this agent (Jiménez-Arribas *et al.*, 2001). If selective and maintenance pressures are so diverse, the control of this kind of multi-resistance could be an impossible task. Moreover, as the resistance phenotype these regulatory loci confer are unspecific, even new, completely unrelated antibiotics, might be less active against such mutants (contrasting with multi-resistance due to the accumulation of specific resistance genes in a single cell or genetic element).

References

Amábile-Cuevas, C.F. and Demple, B. 1991. Molecular characterization of the *soxRS* genes of *Escherichia coli*: two genes control a superoxide stress regulon. Nucleic Acids Res. 19: 4479-4484.

Amábile-Cuevas, C.F. and Fuentes, A.M. 1996. Bacterial regulated responses resulting in antibiotic resistance. In: Antibiotic Resistance: From Molecular Basics To Therapeutic Options. C.F. Amábile-Cuevas, eds. RG Landes/Chapman & Hall, Austin/New York. p. 57-72.

Andersen, J., Forst, S.A., Zhao, K. and Otro, O. 1989. The function of *micF* RNA: *micF* RNA is a major factor in the thermal regulation of OmpF protein in *Escherichia coli*. J. Biol. Chem. 264: 17961-17970.

Ariza, R.R., Cohen, S.P., Bachhawat, N. and Demple, B. 1994. Repressor mutations in the *marRAB* operon that activate oxidative stress genes and multiple antibiotic resistance in *Escherichia coli*. J. Bacteriol. 176: 143-148.

Ariza, R.R., Li, Z., Ringstad, N. and Demple, B. 1995. Activation of multiple antibiotic resistance and binding of stress-inducible promoters by *Escherichia coli* Rob protein. J. Bacteriol. 177: 1655-1661.

Barbosa, T.M. and Levy, S.B. 2000. Differential expression of over 60 chromosomal genes in *Escherichia coli* by constitutive expression of MarA. J. Bacteriol. 182: 3467-3474.

Benov, L. and Fridovich, I. 1996. Functional significance of the Cu,ZnSOD in *Escherichia coli*. Arch. Biochem. Biophys. 327: 249-253.

Bradley, T.M., Hidalgo, H., Leautaud, V., Ding, H. and Demple, B. 1997. Cysteine-to-alanine replacements in the *Escherichia coli* SoxR protein and the role of the [2Fe-2S] centers in transcriptional activation. Nucleic Acids Res. 25: 1469-1475.

Braus, G., Argast, M. and Beck, C.F. 1984. Identification of additional genes on transposon Tn*10*: *tetC* and *tetD*. J. Bacteriol. 160: 504-509.

Demple, B. and Amábile-Cuevas, C.F. 1991. Redox redux: the control of oxidative stress responses. Cell 67: 837-839.

Ding, H., Hidalgo, E. and Demple, B. 1997. The redox state of the [2Fe-2S] clusters in SoxR protein regulates its activity as a transcription factor. J. Biol. Chem. 271: 33173-33175.

Fee, J.A. 1991. Regulation of *sod* genes in *Escherichia coli*: relevance to superoxide dismutase function. Mol. Microbiol. 5: 2599-2610.

Fuentes, A.M. and Amábile-Cuevas, C.F. 1997. Mercury induces multiple antibiotic resistance in *Escherichia coli* through activation of SoxR, a redox-sensing regulatory protein. FEMS Microbiol. Lett. 154: 385-388.

Fuentes, A.M., Díaz-Mejía, J.J., Maldonado-Rodríguez, R. and Amábile-Cuevas, C.F. 2001. Differential activities of SoxR protein of *Escherichia coli*: SoxS is not required for gene activation under iron deprivation. FEMS Microbiol. Lett. 201: 271-275.

Gambino, L., Gracheck, S.J. and Miller, P.F. 1993. Overexpression of the MarA positive regulator is sufficient to confer multiple antibiotic resistance in *Escherichia coli*. J. Bacteriol. 175: 2888-2894.

George, A.M. and Levy, S.B. 1983a. Amplifiable resistance to tetracycline, chloramphenicol, and other antibiotics in *Escherichia coli*: involvement of a non-plasmid-determined efflux of tetracycline. J. Bacteriol. 155: 531-540.

George, A.M. and Levy, S.B. 1983b. Gene in the major cotransduction gap of *Escherichia coli* K-12 linkage map required for the expression of chromosomal resistance to tetracycline and other antibiotics. J. Bacteriol. 155: 541-548.

Giraud, E., Cloeckaert, A., Kerboeuf, D. and Chaslus-Dancla, E. 2000. Evidence for active efflux as the primary mechanism of resistance to ciprofloxacin in *Salmonella enterica* serovar Typhimurium. Antimicrob. Agents Chemother. 44: 1223-1228.

Greenberg, J.T., Chou, J.H., Monach, P.A. and Demple, B. 1991. Activation of oxidative stress genes by mutations at the *soxQ/cfxB/marA* locus of *Escherichia coli*. J. Bacteriol. 173: 4433-4439.

Greenberg, J.T., Monach, P., Chou, J.H., Josephy, P.D. and Demple, B. 1990. Positive control of a global antioxidant defense regulon activated by superoxide-generating agents in *Escherichia coli*. Proc. Natl. Acad. Sci. U.S.A. 87: 6181-6185.

Gruer, M.J. and Guest, J.R. 1994. Two genetically-distinct and differentially-regulated aconitases (AcnA and AcnB) in *Escherichia coli*. Microbiology 140: 2531-2541.

Harder, K.J., Nikaido, H. and Matsuhashi, M. 1981. *Escherichia coli* that are resistant to certain beta-lactam compounds lack the *ompF* porin. Antimicrob. Agents Chemother. 20: 549-552.

Hassett, D.J. and Cohen, M.S. 1989. Bacterial adaptation to oxidative stress: implications for pathogenesis and interaction with phagocytic cells. FASEB J. 3: 2574-2582.

Hidalgo, E., Bollinger, J.M., Bradley, T.M., Walsh, C.T. and Demple, B. 1995. Binuclear [2Fe-2S] clusters in the *Escherichia coli* SoxR protein and the role of the metal centers in transcription. J. Biol. Chem. 270: 20908-20914.

Hidalgo, E. and Demple, B. 1994. An iron-sulfur center essential for transcriptional activation by the redox-sensing SoxR protein. EMBO J. 13: 138-146.

Hidalgo, E. and Demple, B. 1996a. Activation of SoxR-dependent transcription *in vitro* by noncatalytic or NifS-mediated assembly of [2Fe-2S] clusters into apo-SoxR. J. Biol. Chem. 271: 7269-7272.

Hidalgo, E. and Demple, B. 1996b. Adaptive responses to oxidative stress: the *soxRS* and *oxyR* regulons. In: Regulation of Gene Expression in *Escherichia coli*. E.C. Lin and A.S. Lynch, eds. R.G. Landes Co., Austin. p. 435-452.

Hidalgo, E., Leautaud, V. and Demple, B. 1998. The redox-regulated SoxR protein acts from a single DNA site as a repressor and an allosteric activator. EMBO J. 17: 2629-2636.

Hooper, D.C., Wolfson, J.S., Souza, K.S. and Otro, O. 1989. Mechanisms of quinolone resistance in *Escherichia coli*: characterization of *nfxB* and *cfxB*, two mutant resistance loci decreasing norfloxacin accumulation. Antimicrob. Agents Chemother. 33: 283-290.

Imlay, K.R.C. and Imlay, J.A. 1996. Cloning and analysis of *sodC*, encoding the copper-zinc superoxide dismutase of *Escherichia coli*. J. Bacteriol. 178: 2564-2571.

Jair, K.-W., Fawcett, W.P., Fujita, N., Ishihama, A. and Wolf, R.E. 1996a. Ambidextrous transcriptional activation by SoxS: requirement for the C-terminal domain of the RNA polymerase alpha subunit in a subset of *Escherichia coli* superoxide-inducible genes. Mol. Microbiol. 19: 307-317.

Jair, K.-W., Martin, R.G., Rosner, J.L., Fujita, N., Ishihama, A. and Wolf, R.E. 1995. Purification and regulatory properties of MarA protein, a transcriptional activator of *Escherichia coli* multiple antibiotic and superoxide resistance promoters. J. Bacteriol. 177: 7100-7104.

Jair, K.-W., Yu, X., Skarstad, K., Thöny, B., Fujita, N., Ishihama, A. and Wolf, R.E. 1996b. Transcriptional activation of promoters of the superoxide and multiple antibiotic resistance regulons by Rob, a binding protein of the *Escherichia coli* origin of chromosomal replication. J. Bacteriol. 178: 2507-2513.

Jiménez-Arribas, G., Léautaud, V. and Amábile-Cuevas, C.F. 2001. Regulatory locus *soxRS* partially protects *Escherichia coli* against ozone. FEMS Microbiol. Lett. 195: 175-177.

Kargalioglu, Y. and Imlay, J.A. 1994. Importance of anaerobic superoxide dismutase synthesis in facilitating outgrowth of *Escherichia coli* upon entry into an aerobic habitat. J. Bacteriol. 176: 7653-7658.

Kobayashi, K. and Tagawa, S. 1999. Isolation of reductase for SoxR that governs an oxidative response regulon from *Escherichia coli*. FEBS Lett. 451: 227-230.

Koutsolioutsou, A., Martins, E.A., White, D.G., Levy, S.B. and Demple, B. 2001. A *soxRS*-constitutive mutation contributing to antibiotic resistance in a clinical isolate of *Salmonella enterica* (serovar Typhimurium). Antimicrob. Agents Chemother. 45: 38-43.

Li, Z. and Demple, B. 1994. SoxS, an activator of superoxide stress genes in *Escherichia coli*. J. Biol. Chem. 174: 18371-18377.

Liochev, S.I. and Fridovich, I. 1992a. Fumarase C, the stable fumarase of *Escherichia coli*, is controlled by the *soxRS* regulon. Proc. Natl. Acad. Sci. U.S.A. 89: 5892-5896.

Liochev, S.I. and Fridovich, I. 1992b. Superoxide radical in *Escherichia coli*. In: Molecular Biology of Free Radical Scavenging Systems. J.G. Scandalios, eds. Cold Spring Harbor Laboratory Press, Cold Spring Harbor. p. 213-229.

Liochev, S.I., Hausladen, A., Beyer, W.F. and Fridovich, I. 1994. NADPH:ferredoxin oxidoreductase acts as a paraquat diaphorase and is a member of the *soxRS* regulon. Proc. Natl. Acad. Sci. U.S.A. 91: 1328-1331.

Livermore, D.M. 2002. Multiple mechanisms of antimicrobial resistance in *Pseudomonas aeruginosa*: our worst nightmare? Clin. Infect. Dis. 34: 634-640.

Ma, D., Cook, D.N., Alberti, M., Pon, N.G., Nikaido, H. and Hearst, J.E. 1995. Genes *acrA* and *acrB* encode a stress-induced efflux system of *Escherichia coli*. Mol. Microbiol. 16: 45-55.

Martin, J.P., Colina, K. and Logsdon, N. 1987. Role of oxygen radicals in the phototoxicity of tetracyclines toward *Escherichia coli* B. J. Bacteriol. 169: 2516-2522.

McMurry, L.M., George, A.M. and Levy, S.B. 1994. Active efflux of chloramphenicol in susceptible *Escherichia coli* strains and in multiple-antibiotic-resistant (Mar) mutants. Antimicrob. Agents Chemother. 38: 542-546.

McMurry, L.M., Oethinger, M. and Levy, S.B. 1998. Overexpression of *marA*, *soxS*, or *acrAB* produces resistance to triclosan in laboratory and clinical strains of *Escherichia coli*. FEMS Microbiol. Lett. 166: 305-309.

Miller, P.F., Gambino, L.F., Sulavik, M.C. and Gracheck, S.J. 1994. Genetic relationship between *soxRS* and *mar* loci in promoting multiple antibiotic resistance in *Escherichia coli*. Antimicrob. Agents Chemother. 38: 1773-1779.

Moken, M.C., McMurry, L.M. and Levy, S.B. 1997. Selection of multiple-antibiotic-resistant (*mar*) mutants of *Escherichia coli* by using the disinfectant pine oil: roles of the *mar* and *acrAB* loci. Antimicrob. Agents Chemother. 41:

Nunoshiba, T. and Demple, B. 1993. Potent intracellular oxidative stress exerted by the carcinogen 4-nitroquinoline-N-oxide. Cancer Res. 53: 3250-3252.

Nunoshiba, T. and Demple, B. 1994. A cluster of constitutive mutations affecting the C-terminus of the redox-sensitive SoxR transcriptional activator. Nucleic Acids Res. 22: 2958-2962.

Nunoshiba, T., deRojas-Walker, T., Tannenbaum, S.R. and Demple, B. 1995. Roles of nitric oxide in inducible resistance of *Escherichia coli* to activated murine macrophages. Infect. Immun. 63: 794-798.

Nunoshiba, T., deRojas-Walker, T., Whishnok, J.S., Tannenbaum, S.R. and Demple, B. 1993a. Activation by nitric oxide of an oxidative-stress response that defends *Escherichia coli* against activated macrophages. Proc. Natl. Acad. Sci. USA 90: 9993-9997.

Nunoshiba, T., Hidalgo, E., Amábile-Cuevas, C.F. and Demple, B. 1992. Two-stage control of an oxidative stress regulon: the *Escherichia coli* SoxR protein triggers redox-inducible expression of the *soxS* regulatory gene. J. Bacteriol. 174: 6054-6060.

Nunoshiba, T., Hidalgo, E., Li, Z. and Demple, B. 1993b. Negative autoregulation by the *Escherichia coli* SoxS protein: a dampening mechanism for the *soxRS* redox stress response. J. Bacteriol. 175: 7492-7494.

Oethinger, M., Kern, W.V., Jellen-Ritter, A.S., McMurry, L.M. and Levy, S.B. 2000. Ineffectiveness of topoisomerase mutations in mediating clinically significant fluoroquinolone resistance in *Escherichia coli* in the absence of the AcrAB efflux pump. Antimicrob. Agents Chemother. 44: 10-13.

Park, S.-J. and Gunsalus, R.P. 1995. Oxygen, iron, carbon, and superoxide control of the fumarase *fumA* and *fumC* genes of *Escherichia coli*: role of the *arcA*, *fnr*, and *soxR* gene products. J. Bacteriol. 177: 6255-6262.

Pepe, C.M., Suzuki, C., Laurie, C. and Simons, R.W. 1997. Regulation of the "*tetCD*" genes of transposon Tn*10*. J. Mol. Biol. 270: 14-25.

Pomposiello, P.J., Bennik, M.H.J. and Demple, B. 2001. Genome-wide transcriptional profiling of the *Escherichia coli* responses to superoxide stress and sodium salicylate. J. Bacteriol 183: 3890-3902.

Privalle, C.T., Kong, S.E. and Fridovich, I. 1993. Induction of manganese-containing superoxide dismutase in anaerobic *Escherichia coli* by diamide and 1,10-phenanthroline: sites of transcriptional regulation. Proc. Natl. Acad. Sci. USA 90: 2310-2314.

Putman, M., van Veen, H.W. and Konings, W.N. 2000. Molecular properties of bacterial multidrug transporters. Microbiol. Mol. Biol. Rev. 64: 672-693.

Randall, L.P. and Woodward, M.J. 2001. Multiple antibiotic resistance (*mar*) locus in *Salmonella enterica* serovar Typhimurium DT104. Appl. Environ. Microbiol. 67: 1190-1197.

Rosner, J.L. 1985. Nonheritable resistance to chloramphenicol and other antibiotics induced by salicylates and other chemotactic repellants in *Escherichia coli* K-12. Proc. Natl. Acad. Sci. U.S.A. 82: 8771-8774.

Rosner, J.L. and Slonczewski, J.L. 1994. Dual regulation of *inaA* by the multiple antibiotic resistance (Mar) and superoxide (SoxRS) stress response systems of *Escherichia coli*. J. Bacteriol. 176: 6262-6269.

Roualt, T.A. and Klausner, R.D. 1996. Iron sulfur clusters as biosensors of oxidants and iron. Trends Biochem. Sci. 21: 174-177.

Sellers, V.M., Johnson, M.K. and Dailey, H.A. 1996. Function of the [2Fe-2S] cluster in mammalian ferrochelatase: a possible role as a nitric oxide sensor. Biochemistry 35: 2699-2704.

Webber, M.A. and Piddock, L.J.V. 2001. Absence of mutations on *marRAB* or *soxRS* in *acrB*-overexpressing fluoroquinolone-resistant clinical and veterinary isolates of *Escherichia coli*. Antimicrob. Agents Chemother. 45: 1550-1552.

Wu, J. and Weiss, B. 1991. Two divergently transcribed genes, *soxR* and *soxS*, control a superoxide response regulon of *Escherichia coli*. J. Bacteriol. 173: 2864-2871.

Zheng, M., Doan, B., Schneider, T.D. and Storz, G. 1999. OxyR and soxRS regulation of *fur*. J. Bacteriol. 181: 4639-4643.

From: *Multiple Drug Resistant Bacteria*
Edited by: Carlos F. Amábile-Cuevas

Chapter 5

Biofilms and Bacterial Multi-Resistance

Peter Gilbert, Andrew McBain and Alexander H. Rickard

Abstract

Microbial biofilm has become inexorably linked with man's failure to control them by treatment regimes that are effective against suspended bacteria. This failure has been related to a localised concentration of bacteria and their extracellular products (exopolymers and extracellular enzymes), that moderates the access of treatment agents and starves the more deeply placed cells. Biofilms, therefore present gradients of physiology, and of concentration for the imposed treatment agent, where small sub-populations sometimes survive inimical treatments, and death is generally delayed for the least susceptible cells. Such cells must either possess innate insensitivity to a wide variety of treatment agents or they must adopt resistant phenotypes during the sub-lethal phases of treatment. Sub-lethal exposure to chemical anti-microbial agents has been shown to induce expression of multi-drug efflux pumps and to favour efflux mutants within populations. Since not all anti-microbial agents are substrates for energetic efflux, then this cannot provide a singular explanation of biofilm-resistance. Indeed, it is the diversity of action mechanisms within those agents towards which biofilms are resistant that makes singular explanations of resistance phenomena difficult. Recently, a number of concepts have been introduced that impinge greatly upon this area of research. The first of these introduces the concept that sub-lethally damaged micro-organisms undergo apoptosis (suicide) before the levels of damage achieve critical dimension, and that a small proportion of cells within any population is mutated such that they do not. This provides a common mechanism of death for a wide-variety of treatment agents and thereby the possibility of common resistance mechanisms that may be of particular advantage within biofilm communities. The second recognises that materials lost from damaged cells may act as signals, *alarmones* that induce a less susceptible phenotype in the vicinity of the inimical stress. These and the more classical explanations of the resistance of microbial biofilms will be presented and discussed in the light of up-to-date literature.

Introduction

The earliest associations between the growth of bacteria as biofilms and the demonstration of multi-drug resistance were made in the early 1980's and stemmed from the clinic (Gristina and Costerton, 1985; Nickel *et al.*, 1985). At this time the use of implanted medical devices was in its ascendancy. In some instances of implantation, episodes of bacteraemia were reported that were responsive to antibiotic treatment and linked to isolates with minimum inhibitory concentrations that were below defined resistance thresholds, but which recurred shortly after the treatment was stopped. Infections could only be resolved when the implanted devices had been removed. The devices were subsequently found to harbour the implicated pathogen as a biofilm, (Gristina *et al.*, 1987, 1989; Evans and Holmes, 1987; Costerton *et al.*, 1987; Bisno and Waldvogel, 1989). At this time examples of bacterial resistance towards aggressive biocidal treatments were also being related to the attached, biofilm mode of growth (Costerton and Lashen, 1984; McCoy *et al.*, 1986a,1986b; Favero *et al.*, 1983). The range of anti-microbial molecules to which biofilm populations appeared to be resistant was considerable and embraced virtually all of the clinically deployed antibiotics, oxidising biocides such as the isothiazolones, the halogens, quaternary ammonium compounds, biguanides and phenolics.

Generally, failure of microorganisms to succumb to antimicrobial treatments arises through an inherent insusceptibility to the agents employed. This may be through the acquisition of resistance, by mutation or gene transfer, or through the emergence of pre-existing, but unexpressed, resistant phenotypes. With few exceptions biofilms are enveloped within extensive extracellular polymeric matrices (glycocalyx). These not only cement and immobilise the cells with respect to one another (Sutherland, 2001), but they also trap molecules and ions of environmental and microbial origin (Sutherland, 2001). Since the diversity of agents towards which biofilms were resistant was vast, and encompassed a variety of action mechanism, then the intuitive explanation of this recalcitrance was that such agents had been prevented from reaching the target cells.

The Glycocalyx and Resistance

The glycocalyx cannot be considered as homogeneous, rather it varies in hydration with depth and, in mixed species communities, provides a mosaic of enveloped microcolonies each being surrounded by polymers with different physico-chemical properties. At the interface of such mosaics, mixed colloidal solutions comprised of the juxtaposed polymers, are substantially different from those of the component polymers. Adsorption sites within the matrix serve to anchor extracellular enzymes from the producer organisms, and will also actively concentrate ionic materials from the bulk fluid phase, and secondary metabolites (including some cell-cell signalling substances) from the community itself. Immobilised enzymes are not only capable of mobilising complex nutrients captured from the fluid phase, but they are also capable of degrading many antibacterial substances. The glycocalyx is therefore able to moderate the micro-environments of each of the individual community members.

The Glycocalyx as a Diffusion Barrier for Antibacterials

Much, but not all, of the resistance characteristics of biofilm communities are lost when these communities are re-suspended and separated from their extracellular products. It is not surprising therefore that many groups of workers have suggested that the glycocalyx acts as a protective umbrella that physically prevents the access of antimicrobials to the underlying cells. In this respect many early studies of antibiotic action against biofilms attributed their ineffectiveness, purely and simply, to the presence of a diffusion barrier (Slack and Nichols, 1981, 1982; Costerton *et al.*, 1987; Suci *et al.,* 1994). Such universal explanations have been refuted (Gordon *et al.,* 1988; Nichols *et al.,* 1988, 1989) since reductions in the diffusion coefficients of antibiotics such as tobramycin and cefsulodin, within biofilms or microcolonies, are insufficient to account for the observed changes in their activity.

The Glycocalyx as a Penetration Barrier against Antibiotic Penetration

The extent of retardation of antibiotic diffusion, alone, is insufficient to account for reduced susceptibility of biofilms. If, however, the antimicrobial agents are strongly charged (*i.e.*, tobramycin) or reactive chemically (*i.e.*, halogens / peroxygens), then they will be chemically quenched within the matrix during diffusion, either by adsorption to the charged matrix (Hoyle and Costerton, 1991; Hoyle *et al.,* 1992) or by chemical reactions that quench the agent (Huang *et al.*, 1995; Stewart *et al.*, 1998). In such instances, whether or not the exopolymeric matrix constitutes a physical barrier to the antimicrobial depends not only upon the nature of the agent, but also upon the binding capacity of the polymeric matrix, the levels of agent used therapeutically (Nichols, 1993), the distribution of biomass and local hydrodynamics (DeBeer *et al.*, 1994), together with the rate of turnover of the microcolony relative to antibiotic diffusion rate (Kumon *et al.*, 1994). For antibiotics such as cefsoludin such effects are therefore likely to be minimal (Nichols *et al.*, 1988, 1989), but they will be high for positively charged antibiotics such as the aminoglycosides (Nichols *et al.*, 1988) and biocides such as polymeric biguanides (Gilbert *et al.,* 2001). In all instances, diffusion would only be slowed rather than halted. If the underlying cells were to be protected through adsorptive losses then the number of adsorption sites must be sufficient to deplete the available drug. This is an unlikely situation in soft tissue infections, but is possible in confined body compartments such as the lung and brain.

Enzyme-mediated Reaction-Diffusion Resistance to Antibiotics

The reaction-diffusion-limitation properties of the glycocalyx (above) could be significantly enhanced if it contained extracellular enzymes that were capable of degrading the diffusing substrate. In this respect a catalytic (*i.e.*, enzymatic) reaction could lead to severe antibiotic-penetration failure (Stewart, 1996), provided that the turnover of substrate by the enzyme was sufficiently rapid. In such respects, it is significant that the expression of hydrolytic enzymes, such as β-lactamases, is induced/de-repressed in adherent populations and in those exposed to sub-lethal concentrations of imipenem and/or piperacillin (Lambert *et al.*, 1993; Giwercman *et al.*, 1991). These enzymes become trapped and concentrated within the biofilm matrix and are able to further impede the penetration and action of susceptible antibiotics. Similarly the inactivation of formaldehyde can be mediated by the enzymes formaldehyde lyase and formaldehyde dehydrogenase (Sondossi *et al.*, 1985). In mixed community biofilms, the production of neutralising enzymes by a single community member will confer protection upon the remainder (Elkins *et al.*, 1999; Hassett *et al.*, 1999; Stewart *et al.*, 2000).

With the exception of those specific examples that involve drug-inactivating enzymes then an invocation of the properties of the glycocalyx has proven insufficient to explain the whole panoply of resistance displayed by the communities (Brown *et al.*, 1988; Gilbert *et al.*, 1990; Brown *et al.*, 1990). Accordingly, physiological changes in the biofilm cells, mediated through the induction of slow growth rates and starvation-responses, together with induction of separate attachment-specific, drug-resistant physiologies have been considered as further mediators of biofilm resistance (Gilbert and Allison, 2000, Allison *et al.*, 2000).

Physiological Status In Biofilm As A Moderator of Resistance

At any given time, a plethora of phenotypes is represented within a biofilm population that reflects the chemical heterogeneity within the glycocalyx and the imposition, through cellular metabolism, of chemical, electrochemical and gaseous gradients. Since it is long established that the susceptibility of bacterial cells towards antibiotics and biocides is profoundly affected by their nutrient status and growth rate then this might substantially affect the susceptibility of the biofilm community. These effects are in addition to those of temperature, pH and prior-exposure to sub-effective concentrations of the agents (Brown and Williams, 1985; Williams, 1988; Brown *et al.*, 1990; Gilbert *et al.*, 1990). Changes in antibiotic susceptibility through phenotypic expression relate not only to growth-rate dependent changes in a variety of cellular components that include membrane fatty-acids, phospholipids and envelope proteins (Gilbert and Brown 1978a,b., Wright and Gilbert, 1987a,b,c; Al-Hiti and Gilbert, 1980; Gilbert and Brown, 1980; Klemperer *et al.*, 1979) but also to the production of extracellular enzymes (Giwercman *et al.*, 1991) and polysaccharides (Govan and Fyfe, 1978). Whilst gradients of growth rate and the manifestation of phenotypic mosaics have been assumed to occur widely within biofilm populations, and to contribute towards the observed recalcitrance (Brown *et al.*, 1988; Brown *et al.*, 1990, Evans *et al.*, 1990a,b), they have only recently been visualised (Wentland *et al.* 1996; Huang *et al.* 1998; Xu *et al.* 1998). Particularly it has been noted that even within monoculture biofilms, grown in laboratory systems, the established physiological gradients are non-uniform and take on the appearance of a mosaic, with pockets of very slow-growing cells juxtaposed with relatively fast growing areas (Xu *et al.*, 2000).

A number of studies have formally associated the interdependence of growth rate and nutrient limitation in biofilms with their antibiotic susceptibility. Ashby *et al.* (1994) calculated ratios of isoeffective concentration (growth inhibition and bactericidal activity) for biofilm and planktonic bacteria for a wide range of antibiotics against cells grown in broth or on urinary catheter discs and that such ratios followed closely those generated between non-growing and actively-growing cultures. With the exception of ciprofloxacin, antibiotic agents that were most effective against non-growing cultures (*i.e.*, imipenem, meropenem) were also the most active against these biofilms. Other workers have used perfused biofilm fermenters (Gilbert *et al.*, 1989; Hodgson *et al.*, 1995) to directly control and study the effects of growth rate within biofilms. Control populations of planktonic cells were generated in chemostat enabling the separate contributions of growth rate, and association within a biofilm to be evaluated. Decreased susceptibility of *Staphylococcus epidermis* to ciprofloxacin (Duguid *et al.*, 1992) and of *Escherichia coli* to tobramycin (Evans *et al.*, 1990b) and the quaternary ammonium biocide, cetrimide (Evans *et al.*, 1990a) could be explained almost exclusively in terms of the local specific growth rate, in that cells resuspended from growth rate controlled biofilms and planktonic cells, grown at the same growth rate, possessed virtually identical susceptibilities. In such instances, however, when intact biofilms were treated then the susceptibility was decreased somewhat from that of planktonic and resuspended biofilm cells. This indicated some resistance-benefit associated with of organisation of the cells within an exopolymeric matrix.

Why Chemical and Physiological Gradients Provide Incomplete Explanations to Biofilm Resistance

Stewart (1994), developed mathematical models that incorporated the concepts of metabolism-driven oxygen-gradients, growth-rate dependent killing and the reaction-diffusion properties of the glycocalyx that explained the insusceptibility of *S. epidermidis* biofilms towards various antibiotics. This model was able to accurately predict the reductions in susceptibility within thick biofilms through depletion of oxygen. Since nutrient and gaseous gradients will increase in extent as biofilms thicken and mature, then growth-rate effects, such as these, become more evident in matured biofilms (Anwar *et al.*, 1989, 1990). This probably accounts for reports that aged biofilms are more recalcitrant to antibiotic and biocide treatments than are younger ones (Anwar *et al.*, 1989).

The contribution towards resistance within biofilm communities of reductions in growth rate is profound but as with reaction-diffusion, it cannot explain the totality of the observed resistance (Xu *et al.*, 2000). Physiological gradients depend upon growth and metabolism by cells on the periphery to deplete the nutrients as they diffuse towards the more deeply placed cells. Peripheral cells will therefore have growth rates and nutrient profiles that are similar to those in the planktonic phase. Consequently, these cells will be relatively sensitive to antibiotics and will quickly succumb. Lysis products from such cells will feed survivors within the depths of the biofilm which would, as a consequence, step up their metabolism and growth rate, adopt a more susceptible phenotype, and die (McBain *et al.*, 2000). This phenomenon would occur throughout the biofilm, proceeding inwards from the outside, until the biofilm was completely killed. Should the antibiotic become depleted then the biofilm could re-establish almost as quickly as it was destroyed because of the local abundance of trapped nutrients. Growth-rate related processes might therefore delay the onset of killing in the recesses of a biofilm, but can not confer resistance against sustained exposure to antibiotics. Reaction-diffusion limitation of the access of agent, and the existence of physiological gradients within biofilms, provide explanations for their reduced susceptibility, but neither explanation, separately or together, can explain the observations of sustained resistance towards a diverse array of treatment agents. In order for such resistance to be displayed then the biofilm population must either contain cells with unique resistance physiologies, or the short-tem survivors must adapt to a resistant phenotype during the 'time-window' of opportunity provided by the buffering effects of diffusion and growth rate (*i.e.*, a rapid response to sub-lethal treatment).

Drug Resistant Physiologies

The diversity of agents towards which biofilms have been observed to be resistant, together with the long-term survival, of biofilms in the presence of vast excesses of treatment agent make alternate explanations necessary. Since the biofilm victory over antibiotics is Phyrric then long-term survival might be related to the presence of a small fraction of the population that expresses a highly recalcitrant physiology. Possible physiologies include dormant 'quiescent' cells, expression of efflux pumps, and suicide-less mutants.

Quiescence

Over the last 10 years there has been much speculation concerning the ability of non-sporulating bacteria to adopt spore-like qualities in a quiescent state. Specific growth rates of such cells approach zero (Moyer and Morita, 1989) as they undergo reductive divisions in order to complete the segregation of initiated rounds of chromosome replication (Moyer and Morita, 1989; Novitsky and Morita, 1976, 1977). Such quiescent cells have generally been associated with biofilms in oligotrophic marine environments (Kjelleberg *et al.*, 1982) but are likely also to be the dominant form of bacteria within environments of low nutrient availability (Morita, 1986). Whilst mainly associated with aquatic, Gram-negative bacteria, such quiescence has recently been reported in Gram-positives (Lleo *et al.*, 1998), and would appear to be a universal response to extreme nutrient stress (Matin *et al.*, 1989). This has been termed the general stress response (GSR) and leads to populations of cells that synthesise highly phosphorylated nucleotides ppApp and pppApp (Piggot and Coote, 1976; Rhaese *et al.*, 1975) and become resistant to a wide range of physical and chemical agents (Hengge-Aronis, 1996; Matin *et al.*, 1989). GSR is now thought to account for much of the resistance observed in stationary phase cultures and is induced under conditions of extreme starvation.

Various terms have been adopted to describe such phenotypes, including "resting" (Munro *et al.*, 1989), "quiescent" (Trainor *et al.*, 1999), "ultra-microbacteria" (Novitsky and Morita, 1976) "dormant" (Amy *et al.*, 1983; Lim *et al.*, 1999) and Somnicells (Roszak and Colwell, 1987a). It is also likely that the same phenomena describes the state of viable but non-culturable (VNC) (Barer and Harwood, 1999) since such bacterial cells often fail to produce colonies when transferred directly onto nutrient rich agar. Indeed, when bacteria are collected and plated from oligotrophic environments then there is often a great disparity between the viable and total cell counts obtained (Roszak and Colwell, 1987a,b; Defives *et al.*, 1999). Even within biofilms that are in eutrophic environments, regions exist where nutrients are scarce or even absent. Under such circumstances a small proportion of the cells present within a mature biofilm will be expressing the GSR regulator and will be relatively recalcitrant to inimical treatments. Similar mechanisms have been proposed for the hostile take-over of batch cultures by killer-phenotypes during the stationary phase (Zambrano and Kolter, 1995), induced as part of the GSR in *E. coli*. This can lead to a phenotype that is not only more competitive in its growth than non-stressed cells, but which can also directly bring about the death of non-stressed ones (Zambrano *et al.*, 1993). Whilst such phenomena have been reported in variously grown batch cultures, adoption of a killer phenotype by either the biofilm or émigrés from a biofilm would facilitate colonisation resistance or invasiveness respectively. In this respect the general stress response can be associated with the separate regulation of at least 30 distinct proteins (Zambrano and Kolter, 1995) some of which might be assigned as cell-bound bacteriocins / binding-receptors.

The *rpoS*-encoded sigma factor σ^s is a cental regulator within a complex network of stationary phase responsive genes in *E. coli* (Hennge-Arronis, 1996) whereas in *P. aeruginosa* it appears that at least two sigma factors RpoS and AlgU, and also the density-dependent cell-cell signalling systems orchestrate such responses (Foley *et al.*, 1999). Indeed there is a hierarchical link between *n*-acyl homoserine lactones and *rpoS* expression (Latifi *et al.*, 1996) which might specifically induce the quiescent state at locations within a biofilm where signals accumulate and where nutrients are most scarce. In such respects it was elegantly demonstrated by Foley *et al.* (1999) that the GSR response regulator *rpoS* was highly expressed in all of 19 *P. aeruginosa* infected sputum samples taken from cystic fibrosis patients.

Efflux Pumps

An increasingly observed and appreciated resistance mechanism is the expression and possible over-production of multidrug efflux pumps (Nikaido, 1996). In Gram-negative and Gram-positive bacteria the expression of such pumps is induced through sub-lethal exposure to a broad-range of agents (George and Levy, 1983; Ma *et al.*, 1993). These agents include not only small hydrophilic antibiotics but also other xenobiotics such as pine oil, salicylate and triclosan (Miller and Sulavick, 1996; Moken *et al.,* 1997). Efflux pumps are present and operate in many Gram-negative organisms, and may be plasmid or chromosomally encoded (Nikaido, 1996). In addition, multidrug efflux pumps *qacA - G* also contribute to biocide tolerance in Gram positive *Staphylococcus aureus* (Rouch *et al.* 1990). Sublethal exposure of *P. aeruginosa mexAB* mutants to many antimicrobials can select for cells that hyper-express an alternate efflux pump *mexCD* (Chuanchuen *et al.,* 2000; 2001). This highlights the multiplicity of efflux genes and their highly conserved nature.

Several attempts have been made to group efflux pumps into families (Griffith *et al.*, 1992) and to predict structure and function of the proteins themselves (Saier, 1994; Johnson and Church, 1999). Four superfamilies of efflux pumps have been recognised (Saier and Paulsen, 2001). Although the families share no significant sequence identity, substrate specificity is often shared between them (Paulsen *et al.*, 1996). All the efflux superfamiles, however, contain pumps that are specific for single agents together with broader-specificity multidrug efflux pumps which are capable of expelling a broad range of structurally unrelated antibiotics and disinfectants from the cells. Any type of efflux pump may be involved primarily with the expulsion of endogenous metabolites or, alternatively, may be involved primarily with the efflux of chemotherapeutic agents. Indeed, it is probable that these exporters were originally developed to expel endogenous metabolites, but that a coincident ability to exclude harmful substances has proven to be a desirable survival strategy which has been selected for, and incorporated, by almost every known genus and species of bacterium.

Most notable amongst the multidrug resistance operons are the *mar* and *acrAB* efflux pumps (George and Levy, 1983; Ma *et al.*, 1993). The *mar* locus of *E. coli* was the first mechanism found to be involved in the chromosomally encoded, intrinsic resistance of Gram-negative bacteria to multiple drugs. Homologues have since been described in many Gram-negative bacteria. Moken *et al.* (1997) and McMurry *et al.* (1998b) have shown that mutations causing over-expression of *marA* or *acrAB* are associated with exposure and reduced susceptibility towards a wide range of chemicals and antibiotics. The importance of *mar* and efflux systems generally would, however, be far greater if it were induced by growth as a biofilm *per se*. In such instances a generalised efflux of toxic agents would provide explanation of the ubiquitous observation of resistance, regardless of the treatment agent, and would be conferred upon the cells prior to exposure.

Ciprofloxacin exposure does not induce the expression of *mar* or *acrAB* in *E. coli* but such expression will confer limited protection against this agent. Exposure to ciprofloxacin of biofilms comprised of wild-type, constitutive and *mar*-deleted strains ought to evaluate whether or not such genes were up-regulated in unexposed biofilm communities. Maira-Litran *et al.* (2000a) perfused biofilms of such *E. coli* strains for 48 h with various concentrations of ciprofloxacin. These experiments, whilst demonstrating reduced susceptibility in the *mar* constitutive strain showed little or no difference between wild-type and *mar*-deleted strains (Maira-Litran *et al.*, 2000a). Similar experiments using biofilms constructed from strains in which the efflux pump *acrAB* was either deleted or constitutively expressed (Maira-Litran *et al.*, 2000b) showed the *acrAB* deletion to not significantly affect susceptibility over that of the wild-type strain.

Clearly neither *mar* nor *acrAB* is induced by sub-lethal treatment of biofilms with other than with inducer substances. On the other hand, constitutive expression of *acrAB* protected the biofilm against low concentrations of ciprofloxacin. Studies conducted in continuous culture with a *lacZ* reporter gene fused to *marO_{II}* showed, *mar* expression to be inversely related to specific growth rate (Maira-Litran *et al.*, 2000b). Thus, following exposure of biofilms to sub-lethal levels of β-lactams, tetracyclines and salicylates *mar* expression will be greatest within the depths of the biofilm, where growth rates are suppressed, and might account of the long-term survival of the community when exposed to inducer molecules. Another recent study of efflux in biofilms showed that expression of the major multidrug efflux pumps of *P. aeruginosa* actually decreased as the biofilm developed. Also, although expression was greatest in the depths of the biofilm, experiments with deletion mutants showed that none of the multidrug efflux pumps were contributing to the general, increased resistance to antibiotics exhibited by the biofilm (DeKievet *et al.*, 2001).

Suicide-Less Mutants

It is becoming increasingly clear that many bacterial species are capable of undergoing apoptosis or programmed cell death (Jensen and Gerdes, 1995; Naito *et al.*, 1995; Yarmolinsky, 1995; Engelberg-Kulka and Glaser, 1999; Lewis, 2000). Bacterial programmed cell death is not advantageous if these organisms exist primarily in a planktonic mode. Indeed, suicide is never beneficial to the individual cell but if one considers eukaryote cells then it is often a highly evolved mechanism displayed within tissues. Since bacterial biofilm populations are arguably functional tissues (Costerton *et al.*, 1994) and may be regarded as proliferating entities (Caldwell and Costerton, 1996), then it is highly probable that programmed cell death is an important factor to the biofilm mode of growth.

A recent hypothesis concerning the recalcitrance of biofilm relates to the potential of stressed or damaged bacterial cells to undergo programmed cell death. Lewis (2000, 2001) has suggested that the death of bacteria following treatments with bactericidal agents results not from direct action of the agent, but from a programmed suicide mechanism and cellular lysis (Black *et al.*, 1991; Moyed and Bertrand, 1983). If this is the case, then cells subjected to different treatment agents with different mechanisms of action may well die from a common process. A singular mechanism of death allows us to speculate that singular mechanisms enhance resistance towards and survival from inimical treatments.

If an entire population of cells underwent programmed cell-death simultaneously, as the result of a sub-lethal exposure of anti-microbial, then little benefit would be derived. It is essential that a small proportion of the population be able to avoid such a response and ultimately be responsible for the survival and recovery of the community. It is equally important that this trait of selfishness is not retained in the resultant clones.

The biocide literature of the last 50 years has been punctuated with reports of low-level, persistent survival of anti-microbial treatments (tailing) where the agent has not been quenched and where the survivors do not demonstrate resistance when re-cultured or cloned (Bigger, 1944). Whilst this might relate to a sub-population of cells that are quiescent (described above), the recent evidence suggests that such cells, rather than being resistant to the agent (Koch, 1987) might be defective in programmed cell death (Brooun *et al.*, 2000). Following removal of an inimical stress, these damaged persistors would grow rapidly in the presence of nutrients released from their lysed community partners and the community would become restored. It is also postulated that biofilm populations are enriched in 'persistor' cells, possibly as a biofilm-specific phenotype. Due to their protection, from immune responses or predation, within the biofilm these cells would survive treatment phases and proliferate in the post-treatment phase (Lewis, 2000; 2001). This would engender considerable recalcitrance within the biofilm community.

Selection / Induction of Resistant Phenotypes Through Sub-Effective Treatments

The basic tenet of Darwinian theories of evolution is that all populations are genetically diverse and that continued exposure to any environmental stress will lead to an expansion of the most suited genotype / phenotype. This is particularly the case for mixed community biofilms but applies equally to planktonic cultures of bacteria. Exposure of a population to sub-lethal concentrations of biocides and antibiotics will therefore enrich for the least susceptible clones. Equally, death and lysis of a sub-set of cells might confer resistance properties upon the residual.

Selection of Less Susceptible Clones

It has long been demonstrated that pure cultures of bacteria can be 'trained' to become more tolerant of antibiotics (Brown *et al.*, 1969) and biocides (Maclehose *et al.*, 2001; Brozel and Cloete., 1993; McMurry *et al.*,1998a). In such experiments cultures are either grown in liquid media that contain concentrations of agent that are below the MIC or they are streaked onto gradient plates that incorporate the agent. At each step in the process the MIC is re-determined and the process repeated. In such a fashion it is relatively easy to select for populations of bacteria that have significantly increased MIC values towards the selected agents. In some instances the changes in MIC are enough to render the cells resistant to normal treatment regimes. Where groups of agents have common biochemical targets then it is possible for selection by one agent to confer cross-resistance to a third party agent (Chuanchuen *et al.*, 2001).

Such 'resistance-training' has for many years been regarded as artefactual, since it is difficult to imagine a set of circumstances in the Real-World where bacteria will be exposed to gradually increasing concentrations of an inhibitory agent over a prolonged period. Repeated, sub-lethal treatment of biofilms, in the environment and in infection, however, provide one situation where this might happen (McBain *et al.*, 2000). As with any process involving changes in susceptibility to inimical agents the nature of the genotype / phenotype selected reflects changes in the biocidal / inhibitory targets, the adoption of alternate physiologies that circumvent the target or to changes in drug access. The latter might be through modifications in the cell envelope (Brown *et al.,* 1990, Gilbert *et al.,* 1990) or it might reflect active efflux mechanisms (Levy, 1992). Generally, there is a fitness cost associated with such adaptation but this appears to decrease with continued exposure to the stress (Levin *et al.*, 2000). In such a fashion it has recently been shown that sub-lethal exposure of Gram-negative bacteria to the commonly deployed antibacterial agent triclosan, selects for cells that are mutated in the *fabI* gene (McMurry *et al.*, 1998a). This encodes for the enoyl reductase associated with fatty acid biosynthesis (Heath and Rock, 1995). Similarly exposure of pseudomonads to sub-lethal concentrations of isothiazolones causes the repression of an outer membrane protein *ompT* thought to facilitate uptake of this biocide in normal cells (Brozel and Cloete, 1994).

Mutations that increase the expression of multi-drug efflux pumps result in elevated levels of resistance to a wide range of agents. Thus, mutations in the *mar* operon increase the expression of the *acrAB* efflux pump in *E.* coli (McMurry *et al.*, 1998b) and mutations in the *mexAB* operon of *P. aeruginosa* leads to significant over-expression (Rella and Haas, 1982). It must be borne in mind that the primary function of energetic efflux is to defend the cell against naturally occurring environmental toxicants (Miller and Sulavick, 1996). Efflux is often non-specific and equivalent to an emetic 'vomit' response. Cells that efflux permanently will be poor competitors in heterogeneous communities and will not prosper in the absence of the selection stress. Treatment with antimicrobials that act as substrates, but are not themselves inducers (Chuanchuen *et al.*, 2001; Maira-Litran *et al.*, 2000a,b), might lead to a clonal expansion of mutant cells that are constitutive in efflux pump expression. Treatment with agents that are both strong inducers and also substrates (Sundheim *et al.*, 1998; Moken *et al.*, 1997, Thanassi *et al.*, 1995) will confer no selective advantage upon the efflux mutants, but it must be borne in mind that induction of efflux by one agent will confer a broad spectrum of resistance.

Alarmones

The subject of alarmones have recently been discussed to a number of intriguing reviews (Rowbury 2000, 2001a, 2001b). A variety of intracellular molecules, termed alarmones (Bochner *et al.,* 1984), enable cells to respond to the intra-cellular accumulation of chemicals to toxic levels. These are well documented and include the *soxR* and *oxyR* sensing of superoxide and peroxides (Kullik *et al.*, 1995). Even if these inducers were released from those cells that had been targeted and killed by chemical agents, then they are unlikely to modify cells within the vicinity of the damage since they only poorly penetrate healthy cell walls and membranes. A growing body of literature suggests, however, that bacteria can produce constitutively extracellular sensing components that can be converted (activated) into extracellular inducers by certain types of stress. Unlike the intracellular alarmones, these small, readily diffusible molecules can easily reach other unstressed bacteria and induce the expression of tolerance before the recipients of the signal become exposed (Rowbury, 2001a). Such inducible expression of tolerance has been related to the exposure of bacteria to a variety of physical and chemical agents (Rowbury, 2000) and manifest as reduced susceptibility towards acids, alkali, alkylating agents, electrophiles, oxidising agents and heat (Samson and Cairns, 1977; Demple and Halbrook, 1983; Mackey and Derrick, 1986).

To date there have been no publications relating extracellular alarmones to the resistance of biofilm communities. However, it is tempting to postulate that such extracellular sensors are retained within the biofilm matrix and act as an early warning system of the arrival of toxic environmental agents. Therefore, cells deep within the biofilm would sense an impending threat during chemical treatments and adopt a resistant phenotype. Such phenotypes might include the GSR, adoption of a suicide-less frame of mind or indeed the expression of efflux pumps. It is also tempting to suggest however that rather than induce resistance during an inimical treatment alarmones actually awaken quiescent cells post-treatment.

Conclusions

Resistance of microbial biofilms to a wide variety of antimicrobial agents is clearly associated with the organisation of cells within an exopolymer matrix. Such organisation is able to moderate the concentrations of antimicrobial and antibiotics to which the more deeply lying members of the biofilm community are exposed. These cells are typically starved or slow-growing and express stressed phenotypes that may include the expression or up-regulation of efflux pumps. The expressed phenotype of the deeply seated biofilm community reduces their susceptibility to the treatment agents and increases the probability of their being exposed to sub-lethal concentrations of antimicrobial agent. The deeper-lying cells will out survive those at the surface and multiply if the bulk of the treatment agent is depleted or if the exposure is only transient. Thus, at the fringes of action, selection pressures will enrich the populations with the least susceptible genotype. It is possible under such circumstances for repeated chronic exposure to sub-lethal treatments to select for a more resistant population.

Alternative explanations of the resistance of biofilm communities lies with their expression of biofilm-specific phenotypes, that are so significantly different to those of planktonic cells, that the agents developed against the latter fail to operate on cells within the biofilm. Whilst such phenotypes are known to be expressed and might be regulated through quorum sensing mechanisms, they to do not appear to contribute greatly to the susceptibility pattern of individual biofilm cells.

References

Al-Hiti, M.M. and Gilbert, P. 1980. Changes in preservative sensitivity for the USP antimicrobial agents effectiveness test micro-organisms. J. Appl. Bacteriol. 49: 119-26.

Allison, D.G., McBain, A.J. and Gilbert, P. 2000. Microbial biofilms: problems of control. In: Community Structure and Cooperation in Biofilms. H. Lappin-Scott, P. Gilbert, M. Wilson and D. Roberts, eds. Cambridge University Press, Cambridge. p. 309-327.

Amy, P.S., Pauling, C. and Morita, R.Y. 1983. Recovery from nutrient starvation by a marine *Vibrio* sp. Appl. Environ. Microbiol. 45: 1685-1690.

Anwar, H., Dasgupta, M., Lam, K. and Costerton, J.W. 1989. Tobramycin resistance of mucoid *Pseudomonas aeruginosa* biofilm grown under iron limitation. J. Antimicrob. Chemother. 24: 647-655.

Anwar, H., Dasgupta, M.K. and Costerton, J.W. 1990. Testing the susceptibility of bacteria in biofilms to antibacterial agents. Antimicrob. Agents Chemother. 34: 2043-2046.

Ashby, M.J., Neale, J.E., Knott, S.J. and Critchley, I.A. 1994. Effect of antibiotics on non-growing cells and biofilms of *Escherichia coli*. J. Antimicrob. Chemother. 33: 443-452.

Barer, M.R. and Harwood. C.R. 1999. Bacterial viability and culturability. Adv. Microb. Physiol. 41: 93-137.

Bisno, A.L. and Waldvogel, F.A. 1989. Infections associated with indwelling medical devices. American Society for Microbiology, Washington.

Bigger, J.W. 1944. Treatment of Staphylococcal infection with penicillin. Lancet ii: 497-500.

Black, D.S., Kelly, A.J., Mardis, M.J., and Moyed, H.S. 1991. Structure and organization of *htp*, an operon that affects lethality due to inhibition of peptidoglycan or DNA synthesis. J. Bacteriol. 173: 5732-5739.

Bochner, B.R., Lee, P.C., Wilson, S.W., Cutler, C.W. and Ames, B.N. 1984. AppppA and related adenylated nucleotides are synthesised as a result of oxidation stress. Cell 37: 227-232.

Brooun, A., Liu, S. and Lewis, K. 2000. A dose-response study of antibiotic resistance in *Pseudomonas aeruginosa* biofilms. Antimicrob. Agents Chemother. 44: 640-646.

Brown, M.R.W. and Williams, P. 1985. Influence of substrate limitation and growth phase on sensitivity to antimicrobial agents. J. Antimicrob. Chemother. 15 (Suppl, A): 7-14.

Brown, M.R., Watkins, W.M. and Foster, J.H. 1969. Step-wise resistance to polymyxin and other agents by *Pseudomonas aeruginosa*. J. Gen. Microbiol. 55: 17-18.

Brown, M.R.W., Allison, D.G. and Gilbert, P. 1988. Resistance of bacterial biofilms to antibiotics: a growth rate related effect. J. Antimicrob. Chemother. 22: 777-789.

Brown, M.R.W., Collier, P.J. and Gilbert, P. 1990. Influence of growth rate on the susceptibility to antimicrobial agents: modification of the cell envelope in batch and continuous culture. Antimicrob. Agents Chemother. 34: 1623-1628.

Brozel, V.S. and Cloete, T.E. 1993. Adaptation of *Pseudomonas aeruginosa* to 2,2'-methylenebis (4-chlorophenol). J. Appl. Bacteriol. 74: 94-99.

Brozel, V.S. and Cloete, T.E. 1994. Resistance of *Pseudomonas aeruginosa* to isothiazolone. J. Appl. Bacteriol. 76: 576-82.

Caldwell, D.E. and Costerton, J.W. 1996. Are bacterial biofilms constrained to Darwin's concept of evolution through natural selection? Microbiologia 12: 347-358.

Chuanchuen, R., Beinlich, K. and Schweitzer, H.P. 2000. Multidrug efflux pumps in *Pseudomonas aeruginosa*. Abstracts Annual Meeting of the American Society for Microbiology, Los Angeles, A31.

Chuanchuen, R., Beinlich, K., Hoang, T.T., Becher, A., Karkhoff-Schweizer, R.R., Schweizer, H.P. 2001. Cross-resistance between triclosan and antibiotics in *Pseudomonas aeruginosa* is mediated by multidrug efflux pumps: exposure of a susceptible mutant strain to triclosan selects *nfxB* mutants overexpressing MexCD-OprJ. Antimicrob. Agents Chemother. 45: 428-432.

Costerton, J.W. and Lashen, E.S. 1984. Influence of biofilm on the efficacy of biocides on corrosion-causing bacteria. Materials Perform. 23: 34-37.

Costerton, J.W., Cheng, K.J., Geesey, G.G., Ladd, T.I., Nickel, J.C., Dasgupta, M. and Marrie, T.J. 1987. Bacterial biofilms in nature and disease. Ann. Rev. Microbiol. 41: 435-464.

Costerton, J.W., Lewandowski, Z., Caldwell, D.E., Korber, D.R. and Lappin-Scott, H.M. 1994. Biofilms: the customized microniche. J. Bacteriol. 176: 2137-2142.

DeBeer, D., Srinivasan, R. and Stewart, P.S. 1994. Direct measurement of chlorine penetration into biofilms during disinfection. Appl. Environ. Microb. 60: 4339-4344.

Defives, C., Guyard, S., Oulare, M.M., Mary, P. and Hornez, J.P. 1999. Total counts, culturable and viable, and non-culturable microflora of a French mineral water: a case study. J. Appl. Microbiol. 86: 1033-1038.

DeKievet, T.R., Parkins, M.D., Gillis, R.J., Srikumar, R., Ceri, H., Poole, K.. and Iglewski, B.H. and Storey, D.G. 2001. Multidrug efflux pumps: expression patterns and contribution to antibiotic resistance in *Pseudomonas aeruginosa* biofilms. Antimicrob. Agents Chemother. 45: 1761-1770.

Demple, B. and Halbrook, J. 1983. Inducible repair of oxidative damage in *Escherichia coli*. Nature 304: 466-468.

Duguid, I.G., Evans, E., Brown, M.R.W. and Gilbert, P. 1992. Growth-rate-independent killing by ciprofloxacin of biofilm-derived *Staphylococcus-epidermidis* - evidence for cell-cycle dependency. J Antimicrob. Chemother. 30: 791-802.

Elkins, J.G., Hassett, D.J., Stewart, P.S., Schweizer, H.P. and McDermott, T.R. 1999. Protective role of catalase in *Pseudomonas aeruginosa* biofilm resistance to hydrogen peroxide. Appl. Environ. Microbiol. 65; 4594-600.

Engelberg-Kulka, H. and Glaser, G. 1999. Addiction modules and programmed cell death and anti-death in bacterial cultures. Ann. Rev. Microbiol. 53: 43-70.

Evans, R.C. and Holmes, C.J. 1987. Effect of vancomycin hydrochloride on *Staphylococcus epidermidis* biofilm associated with silicone elastomer. Antimicrob. Agents Chemother. 31: 889-894.

Evans, D.J., Allison, D.G., Brown, M.R. and Gilbert, P. 1990a. Effect of growth-rate on resistance of gram-negative biofilms to cetrimide. J. Antimicrob. Chemother. 26: 473-478.

Evans, D.J., Brown, M.R., Allison, D.G. and Gilbert, P. 1990b. Susceptibility of bacterial biofilms to tobramycin: role of specific growth rate and phase in the division cycle. J. Antimicrob. Chemother. 25: 585-591.

Favero, M.S., Bond, W.W., Peterson, N.J. and Cook, E.H. 1983. Scanning electron microscopic observations of bacteria resistant to iodophor solutions. In: Proceedings of the International Symposium on Povidone. University of Kentucky, Lexington, USA. p.158-166.

Foley, I., Marsh, P., Wellington, E.M., Smith, A.W. and Brown, M.R. 1999. General stress response master regulator *rpoS* is expressed in human infection: a possible role in chronicity. J. Antimicrob. Chemother. 43: 164-165.

George, A.M. and Levy, S.B. 1983. Amplifiable resistance to tetracycline, chloramphenicol, and other antibiotics in *Escherichia coli*: involvement of a non-plasmid-determined efflux of tetracycline. J. Bacteriol. 155: 531-540.

Gilbert, P. and Allison, D. 2000. Biofilms and their resistance towards antimicrobial agents. In: Dental Plaque Revisited. H. Newman and M. Wilson, eds. Bioline, Cardiff. p 125-143.

Gilbert, P. and Brown, M.R. 1978a. Influence of growth rate and nutrient limitation on the gross cellular composition of *Pseudomonas aeruginosa* and its resistance to 3- and 4-chlorophenol. J. Bacteriol. 133: 1066-1072.

Gilbert, P. and Brown, M.R. 1978b. Effect of R-plasmid RP1 and nutrient depletion on the gross cellular composition of *Escherichia coli* and its resistance to some uncoupling phenols. J. Bacteriol. 133: 1062-1065.

Gilbert, P. and Brown, M.R. 1980. Cell wall-mediated changes in sensitivity of *Bacillus megaterium* to chlorhexidine and 2-phenoxyethanol, associated with growth rate and nutrient limitation. J. Appl. Bacteriol. 48: 223-230.

Gilbert, P., Allison, G.G., Evans, D.J., Handley, P.S. and Brown, M.R.W. 1989. Growth rate control of adherent microbial populations. Appl. Environ. Microbiol. 55: 1308-1311.

Gilbert, P., Collier, P.J. and Brown, M.R.W. 1990. Influence of growth rate on susceptibility to antimicrobial agents: Biofilms, cell cycle, dormancy and stringent response. Antimicrob. Agents Chemother. 34: 1865-1868.

Gilbert, P., Das, J.R., Jones, M., and Allison, D.G. 2001. Assessment of the biocide activity upon various bacteria following their attachment to and growth on surfaces J. Appl. Microbiol. 91: 248-255.

Giwercman, B., Jensen, E.T., Hoiby, N., Kharazmi, A. and Costerton, J.W. 1991. Induction of β-lactamase production in *Pseudomonas aeruginosa* biofilms. Antimicrob. Agents Chemother. 35: 1008-1010.

Gordon, C.A., Hodges, N.A. and Marriot, C. 1988. Antibiotic interaction and diffusion through alginate and exopolysaccharide of cystic fibrosis derived *Pseudomonas aeruginosa*. J. Antimicrob. Chemother. 22: 667-674.

Govan, J.R. and Fyfe, J.A. 1978. Mucoid *Pseudomonas aeruginosa* and cystic fibrosis: resistance of the mucoid from to carbenicillin, flucloxacillin and tobramycin and the isolation of mucoid variants in vitro. J. Antimicrob. Chemother. 4: 233-240.

Griffith, J.K., Baker, M.E., Rouch, D.A., Page, M.G.P., Skurray, R.A., Paulsen, I.T., Chater, K.F., Baldwin, S.A. and Henderson, P.J.F. 1992. Membrane transport proteins: implications of sequence comparisons. Curr. Opinion Cell Biol. 4: 684-695.

Gristina A.G. and Costerton J.W. 1985. Bacterial adherence to biomaterials and tissue. The significance of its role in clinical sepsis. J. Bone Joint Surg. Am. 67: 264-273.

Gristina, A.G., Hobgood, C.D., Webb, L.X. and Myrvik, Q.N. 1987. Adhesive colonisation of biomaterials and antibiotic resistance. Biomaterials 8: 423-426.

Gristina, A.G, Jennings, R.A., Naylor, P.T., Myrvik, Q.N. and Webb, L.X. 1989.Comparative in vitro antibiotic-resistance of surface-colonizing coagulase-negative staphylococci. Antimicrob. Agents Chemother. 33: 813-816.

Hassett, D.J., Elkins, J.G., Ma, J.F. and McDermott, T.R. 1999. *Pseudomonas aeruginosa* biofilm sensitivity to biocides: use of hydrogen peroxide as model antimicrobial agent for examining resistance mechanisms. Methods Enzymol. 310: 599-608.

Heath, R.I. and Rock, C.O. 1995. Enoyl-acyl carrier protein reductase (*fabI*) plays a determinant role in completing cycles of fatty-acid elongation in *Escherichia coli*. J. Biol. Chem. 270: 26538- 26542.

Hengge-Aronis R. 1996. Back to log phase: sigma S as a global regulator in the osmotic control of gene expression in *Escherichia coli*. Mol. Microbiol. 21: 887-893.

Hodgson, A.E., Nelson, S.M., Brown, M.R. and Gilbert, P. 1995. A simple in vitro model for growth control of bacterial biofilms. J. Appl. Bacteriol. 79: 87-93.

Hoyle, B.D., and Costerton, J.W. 1991. Bacterial resistance to antibiotics: the role of biofilms. Prog. Drug. Res. 37: 91-105.

Hoyle. B.D., Wong. C.K.W. and Costerton. J.W. 1992. Disparate efficacy of tobramycin on Ca^{2+}-treated, Mg^{2+}-treated, and Hepes-treated *Pseudomonas aeruginosa* biofilms. Can. J. Microbiol. 38: 1214-1218.

Huang, C.T., Yu, F.P., McFeters, G.A. and Stewart, P.S. 1995. Non-uniform spatial patterns of respiratory activity within biofilms during disinfection. Appl. Environ. Microbiol. 61: 2252-2256.

Huang, C.T., Xu, K.D., McFeters, G.A. and Stewart, P.S. 1998. Spatial patterns of alkaline phosphatase expression within bacterial colonies and biofilms in response to phosphate starvation. Appl. Environ. Microbiol. 64: 1526-1531.

Jensen, R.B. and Gerdes, K. 1995. Programmed cell death in bacteria: proteic plasmid stabilised systems. Mol. Microbiol. 17: 205-210.

Johnson, J.M. and Church, G.M. 1999. Alignment and structure prediction of divergent protein families: periplasmic and outer membrane proteins of bacterial efflux pumps. J. Mol. Biol. 287: 695-715.

Kjelleberg, S., Humphrey, B.A. and Marshall, S.C. 1982. Effects of interphases on small, starved marine bacteria. Appl. Environ. Microbiol. 43: 1166-1172.

Klemperer, R.M., Gilbert, P., Meier, A.M., Cozens, R.M. and Brown, M.R. 1979. Influence of suspending media upon the susceptibility of *Pseudomonas aeruginosa* NCTC 6750 and its spheroplasts to polymyxin B. Antimicrob. Agents. Chemother. 15: 147-151.

Koch A.L. 1987. Similarities and differences of individual bacteria within a clone. In: *Escherichia coli* and *Salmonella*: Cellular and Molecular Biology. F.C. Neidhardt, R.I. Curtiss, J.L. Ingraham, C.C.I. Lin, K.B. Low, B. Magasanik, W.S. Reznikoff, M. Riley, M. Scgaechter, and H.E. Umbarger, eds. American Society for Microbiology, Washington. p. 1640-1651.

Kullik, I., Toledano, M.B., Tartaglia, L.A. and Storz, G. 1995. Mutation analysis of the redox sensitive transcriptional regulator OxyR: regions important for oxidation and transcriptional activation. J. Bact. 177: 1275-1284.

Kumon, H., Tomochika, K-I., Matunaga, T., Ogawa, M. and Ohmori, H. 1994. A sandwich cup method for the penetration assay of antimicrobial agents through *Pseudomonas* exopolysaccharides. Microbiol. Immunol. 38: 615-619.

Lambert, P.A., Giwercman, B. and Hoiby, N. 1993. Chemotherapy of *Pseudomonas aeruginosa* in cystic fibrosis. In: Bacterial biofilms and their control in medicine and industry. J.T. Wimpenny, W.W. Nichols, D. Stickler, and H.M. Lappin-Scott, eds. Bioline, Cardiff. p. 151-153.

Latifi, A., Foglino, M., Tanaka, K., Williams, P. and Lazdunski, A. 1996. A hierarchical quorum-sensing cascade in *Pseudomonas aeruginosa* links the transcriptional activators LasR and RhlR (VsmR) to expression of the stationary-phase sigma factor RpoS. Mol. Microbiol. 21: 1137-1146.

Levin, B.R., Perrot, V. and Walker, N. 2000. Compensatory mutations, antibiotic resistance and the population genetics of adaptive evolution in bacteria. Genetics. 154: 985-997.

Levy, S.B. 1992. Active efflux mechanisms for antimicrobial resisitance. Antimicrob. Agents. Chemother. 36: 695-703.

Lewis, K. 2000. Programmed cell death in bacteria. Microbiol. Mol. Biol. Rev. 64: 503-514.

Lewis, K. 2001. Riddle of biofilm resistance. Antimicrob. Agents Chemother. 45, 999-1007.

Lim, A., Eleuterio, M, Hutter, B., Murugasu-Oei, B. and Dick T. 1999. Oxygen depletion-induced dormancy in *Mycobacterium bovis* BCG. J. Bacteriol. 181: 2252-2256.

Lleo, M.D., Tafi, M.C. and Canepari, P. 1998. Nonculturable *Enterococcus faecalis* cells are metabolically active and capable of resuming active growth. Syst. Appl. Microbiol. 21: 333-339.

Ma, D., Cook, D.N., Alberti, M., Pon, N.G., Nikaido, H. and Hearst, J.E. 1993. Molecular cloning and characterization of *acrAB* and *acrE* genes of *Escherichia coli*. J. Bacteriol. 175: 6299-6313.

Maclehose, H.G., Allison, D.G., Gilbert, P. 2001. Susceptibility of *Pseudomonas* spp. to biocides and antibiotics following chronic sub-inhibitory exposure to biocides. Proceedings of the 101st Annual General Meeting of the American Society for Microbiology.

Mackey, B.M. and Derrick, C.M. 1986. Changes in the heat resistance of *Salmonella typhimurium* during heating at rising temperatures. Lett. Appl. Microbiol. 4: 13-16.

Maira-Litran, T., Allison, D.G., and Gilbert, P. 2000a. An evaluation of the potential role of the multiple antibiotic resistance operon (*mar*) and the multi-drug efflux pump *acrAB* in the resistance of *E. coli* biofilms towards ciprofloxacin. J. Antimicrob. Chemother. 45: 789-795.

Maira-Litran, T., Allison, D.G. and Gilbert, P. 2000b. Expression of the multiple resistance operon (*mar*) during growth of *Escherichia coli* as a biofilm, J. Appl. Microbiol. 88: 243-247.

Matin, A., Auger, E.A.., Blum, P.H. and Schultz, J.E. 1989. Genetic basis of starvation survival in non-differentiating bacteria. Annu. Rev, Microbiol. 43: 293-316.

McBain, A.J., Allison, D.G. and Gilbert, P. 2000. Emerging strategies for the chemical treatment of microbial biofilms Biotechnol. Genet. Eng. Rev. 17: 267-279.

McCoy, W., Ridge, J. and Lashen, E. 1986a. Efficacy of biocides in a laboratory model cooling tower. Material Perform. Aug, 9-14.

McCoy, W., Wireman, J. and Lashen, E. 1986b. Efficacy of methylchloroisothiazolone biocide against *Legeionella pneumophila* in cooling tower water. Chimica. Oggi. 4: 79-83.

McMurry, L.M., Oethinger, M. and Levy. S.B. 1998a. Triclosan targets lipid synthesis. Nature 394: 531-532.

McMurry, L.M., Oethinger, M. and Levy, S.B. 1998b. Over expression of *marA*, *soxS*, or *acrAB* produces resistance to triclosan in laboratory and clinical strains of *Escherichia coli*. FEMS Microbiol. Lett. 166: 305-309.

Miller, P.F. and Sulavick, M.C. 1996. Overlaps and parallels in the regulation of intrinsic multiple antibiotic resistance in *Escherichia coli*. Mol. Microbiol. 21: 441-448.

Moken, M.C., McMurry, L.M. and Levy, S.B. 1997. Selection of multiple-antibiotic-resistant (mar) mutants of *Escherichia coli* by using the disinfectant pine oil: roles of the *mar* and *acrAB* loci. Antimicrob. Agents Chemother. 41: 2770-2772.

Morita, R.Y. 1986. Starvation survival: the normal mode of most bacteria in the ocean,. Proc. 4th Inter. Symp. Microbiol. Ecol. Slovene Soc. Microbiol. p. 242-248.

Moyed, H.S. and Bertrand 1983. *hlpA*, a newly recognised gene of *Escherichia coli* that affects frequency of persistence after inhibition of murein synthesis. J. Bacteriol. 155: 768-775.

Moyer, C.L. and Morita, R.Y. 1989. Effect of growth rate and starvation-survival on the viability and stability of a pshycrophylic marine bacterium. Appl. Environ. Microbiol. 55: 1122-1127.

Munro, P.M., Gauthier, M.J., Breittmayer, V.A. and Bongiovanni, J. 1989. Influence of osmoregulation processes on starvation survival of *Escherichia coli* in seawater. Appl Environ Microbiol. 55: 2017-24.

Naito, T., Kusano, K. and Kobayashi, I. 1995. Selfish behaviour of restriction modification systems. Science 267: 897-899.

Nichols, W.W. 1993. Biofilm permeability to antibacterial agents. In: Bacterial Biofilms and Their Control in Medicine and I ndustry. J. Wimpenny, W.W. Nichols, D. Stickler and H. Lappin-Scott, eds. Bioline, Cardiff. p. 141-149.

Nichols. W.W., Dorrington, S.M., Slack, M.P.E. and Walmsley, H.L. 1988. Inhibition of tobramycin diffusion by binding to alginate. Antimicrob. Agents Chemother. 32: 518-523.

Nichols, W.W., Evans, M.J., Slack, M.P.E. and Walmsley, H.L. 1989. The penetration of antibiotics into aggregates of mucoid and non-mucoid *Pseudomonas aeruginosa*. J. Gen. Microbiol. 135: 1291-1303.

Nickel, J.C., Ruseska, I., Wright, J.B. and Costerton, J.W. 1985. Tobramycin resistance of *Pseudomonas aeruginosa* cells growing as a biofilm on urinary catheter material. Antimicrob. Agents Chemother. 27: 619-24.

Nikaido, H. 1996. Multidrug efflux pumps of Gram-negative bacteria. J. Bacteriol. 178: 5853-5859.

Novitsky, J.A. and Morita, R.Y. 1976. Morphological characterisation of small cells resulting from nutrient starvation of a psychrophilic marine vibrio. Appl. Environ. Microbiol. 32: 617-622.

Novitsky, J.A. and Morita, R.Y. 1977. Survival of a phychrophilic marine vibrio under long-term nutrient starvation. Appl. Environ. Microbiol. 33: 635-641.

Paulsen, I.T., Brown, M.H. and Skurray, R.A. 1996. Proton-dependent multidrug efflux systems. Microbiol. Rev. 60: 575-608.

Piggot, P.J. and Coote, J.G. 1976. Genetic aspects of bacteria enospore formation. Bacterial Rev. 40: 908-962.

Rella, M. and Haas, D. 1982. Resistance of *Pseudomonas aeruginosa* PAO to nalidixic acid and low levels of beta-lactam antibiotics: mapping of chromosomal genes. Antimicrob. Agents Chemother. 22: 242-249.

Rhaese, H., Dichtelmüller, R., Grade, R. and Groscurth, R. 1975. High phosphorylated nucloetides involved in regulation of sporulation in

Bacillus subtilis. In: Spores, VI. P. Gerhardt, R. Costliow and H.L. Sadof, eds. American Society for Microbiology, Washington. p. 335-340.

Roszak, D.B. and Colwell, R.R. 1987a. Metabolic activity of bacterial cells enumerated by direct viable count. Appl. Environ. Microbiol. 53: 2889-2893.

Roszak, D.B. and Colwell, R.R. 1987b. Survival strategies of bacteria in the natural environment. Microbial. Rev. 51: 365-379.

Rouch, D.A., Cram, D.S., Dibernadino, D., Littlejohn, T.G. and Skurray, R.A. 1990. Efflux-mediated antiseptic gene *qacA* from *Staphylococcus aureus*: common ancestry with tetracycline and sugar transport proteins. Mol. Microbiol. 4: 2051-2062.

Rowbury, R.J. 2000. Killed cultures of *Escherichia coli* can protect living organisms from acid stress. Microbiology 146: 1759-1760.

Rowbury, R.J. 2001a. Cross-talk involving extracellular sensors and extracellular alarmones gives early warning to unstressed *Escherichia coli* of impending lethal chemical stress and leads to induction of tolerance responses. J. Appl. Microbiol. 90: 677-695.

Rowbury, R.J. 2001b. Extracellular sensing components and extracellular induction component alarmones give early warning against stress in *Escherichia coli*. Adv. Microb. Physiol. 44: 215-257.

Saier, M.H. 1994. Computer-aided analyses of transport protein sequences: gleaning evidence concerning function, structure, biogenesis and evolution. Microbiol. Rev. 58: 71-93.

Saier, M.H., Paulsen, I.T. 2001. Phylogeny of multidrug transporters. Seminars Cell Developmental Biol. 12: 205-213.

Samson, L. and Cairns, J. 1977. A new pathway for DNA repair in *Escherichia coli*. Nature 267: 281-283.

Slack, M.P.E. and Nichols, W.W. 1981. The penetration of antibiotics through sodium alginate and through the exopolysaccharide of a mucoid strain of *Pseudomonas aeruginosa*. Lancet 11: 502-503.

Slack, M.P.E. and Nichols, W.W. 1982. Antibiotic penetration through bacterial capsules and exopolysaccharides. J. Antimicrob. Chemother. 10: 368-372.

Sondossi, M., Rossmore, H.W. and Wireman, J.W. 1985. Observation of resistance and cross-resistance to formaldehyde and a formaldeyde condensate biocide in *Pseudomonas aeruginosa*. Int. Biodet. Biodeg. 21: 105-106.

Stewart, P.S. 1994. Biofilm accumulation model that predicts antibiotic resistance of *Pseudomonas aeruginosa* biofilms. Antimicrob. Agents Chemother. 38: 1052-1058.

Stewart, P.S. 1996. Theoretical aspects of antibiotic diffusion into microbial biofilms. Antimicrob. Agents Chemoth. 40: 2517-2522.

Stewart, P.S., Grab, L. and Diemer, J.A. 1998. Analysis of biocide transport limitation in an artificial biofilm system. J. Appl. Microb. 85: 495-500.

Stewart, P.S., Roe, F., Rayner, J., Elkins, J.G, Lewandowski, Z., Ochsner, U.A. and Hassett, D.J. 2000. Effect of catalase on hydrogen peroxide penetration into *Pseudomonas aeruginosa* biofilms. Appl. Environ. Microbiol. 66: 836-838.

Suci, P.A., Mittelman, M.W., Yu F.P. and Geesey, G.G. 1994. Investigation of ciprofloxacin penetration into *Pseudomonas aeruginosa* biofilms. Antimicrob. Agents Chemother. 38: 2125-2133.

Sundheim, G., Langsrud, S., Heir, E. and Holck, A.L. 1998. Bacterial resistance to disinfectants containing quaternary ammonium compounds. Int. Biodet. Biodeg. 41: 235-239.

Sutherland, I.W. 2001. The biofilm matrix - an immobilized but dynamic microbial environment. Trends Microbiol. 9: 222-227.

Thanassi, D.G., Suh, G.S. and Nikaido, H. 1995. Role of outer membrane barrier in efflux-mediated tetracycline resistance of *Escherichia coli*. J. Bacteriol. 177: 998-1007.

Trainor, V.C., Udy, R.K., Bremer, P.J. and Cook, G.M. 1999. Survival of *Streptococcus pyogenes* under stress and starvation. FEMS Microbiol. Lett. 176: 421-428.

Wentland, E.J., Stewart, P.S., Huang, C.T. and McFeters, G.A. 1996. Spatial variations in growth rate within *Klebsiella pneumoniae* colonies and biofilm. Biotechnol. Prog. 12: 316-321.

Williams, P. 1988. Role of the cell envelope in bacterial adaptation to growth in vivo in infections. Biochemie 70: 987-1011.

Wright, N.E. and Gilbert, P. 1987a. Antimicrobial activity of n-alkyltrimethylammonium bromides: influence of specific growth rate and nutrient limitation. J. Pharm. Pharmacol. 39: 685-690.

Wright, N.E. and Gilbert, P. 1987b. Influence of specific growth rate and nutrient-limitation upon the sensitivity of *Escherichia coli* towards polymyxin B. J. Antimicrob. Chemother. 20: 303-312.

Wright, N.E. and Gilbert, P. 1987c. Influence of specific growth rate and nutrient limitation upon the sensitivity of *Escherichia coli* towards chlorhexidine diacetate. J. Appl. Bacteriol. 62: 309-314.

Xu, K.D., Stewart, P.S., Xia, F., Huang, C.T. and McFeters, G.A. 1998. Spatial physiological heterogeneity in *Pseudomonas aeruginosa* biofilm is determined by oxygen availability. Appl. Environ. Microbiol. 64: 4035-4039.

Xu, K.D., McFeters, G.A. and Stewart, P.S. 2000. Biofilm resistance to antimicrobial agents. Microbiology. 146: 547-549.

Yarmolinsky, M.B. 1995. Programmed cell death in bacterial populations. Science 267: 836-837.

Zambrano, M. and Kolter, R. 1995. Changes in bacterial cell properties in going from exponential growth to stationary phase. In: Microbial quality assurance: a guide towards relevance and reproducibility of inocula. M.R.W Brown and P. Gilbert, eds. CRC, Boca Raton. p. 21-30.

Zambrano, M., Siegele, D. A., Almiron, M., Tormo, A. and Kolter, R. 1993. Microbial competition: *Escherichia coli* mutants that take over stationary phase culture. Science 259: 1757-1760.

From: *Multiple Drug Resistant Bacteria*
Edited by: Carlos F. Amábile-Cuevas

Chapter 6

Vancomycin Resistant Enterococci and Methicillin Resistant *Staphylococcus Aureus*

Henry S. Fraimow

Abstract

Vancomycin-Resistant Enterococci (VRE) and Methicillin-Resistant *Staphylococcus aureus* (MRSA) have emerged as major nosocomial pathogens with enormous public health significance. VRE initially appeared in the late 1980's. In Europe, emergence of VRE may be due to glycopeptide use in animal feeds and VRE can be found in healthy outpatients, but spread in hospitals is more limited than in the United States. In the U.S., emergence of VRE in hospitals is closely associated with increases in vancomycin use, especially for treatment of MRSA infection, as well as overuse of other antimicrobials. VRE now comprise 10% of hospital enterococcal isolates, with rates up to 25% of isolates from ICU infections. Up to 80-90% of strains of *E. faecium* may be vancomycin resistant. Risks for colonization with VRE include exposure to vancomycin and other antimicrobials, ICU stay, gastrointestinal manipulations and renal failure. Once patients are colonized with VRE, organisms are shed from the gastrointestinal tract for prolonged periods. This has complicated control efforts and has contributed to VRE becoming endemic in chronic care settings. Fortunately, transmission of vancomycin resistance genes from enterococci to other pathogenic organisms is extremely rare. Treatment of VRE is limited by the intrinsic resistance of enterococci and the development of acquired multi-drug resistance, especially in *E. faecium*. Several new antimicrobials, including quinupristin/dalfopristin and linezolid, have been developed for treatment of VRE infections.

MRSA first emerged as a significant public health problem in the 1980s and are now a global issue, although there is geographic variability in the prevalence of MRSA. Up to 70% of *S.aureus* in large U.S. teaching hospitals are methicillin resistant, far above the threshold requiring clinicians to empirically use vancomycin for the treatment of suspected staphylococcal infections. These high prevalence rates have also caused a reappraisal of traditional infection control practices designed to limit the spread of MRSA. MRSA are also seen in community acquired infections in intravenous drug users and patients with indirect hospital contacts, but are also now reported in children and adults with no known risk factors. In hospital settings, antibiotic usage remains the major risk for acquisition of MRSA. Treatment options for MRSA infections are limited by frequent multi-resistance. Vancomycin remains the primary treatment option but is associated with a high clinical failure rate and strains with decreased susceptibility to glycopeptides have also been described. New agents such as quinupristin/dalfopristin and linezolid may be useful for treatment of MRSA infections.

Introduction

The predominant trend in the microbiology of nosocomial infections over the past two decades has been the continued emergence of multi-drug resistant gram-positive pathogens as major causes of hospital acquired infections (Figure 1). Strains of *Staphylococcus aureus* resistant to semi-synthetic penicillins such as methicillin (MRSA) appeared in Europe in 1960 and became a major problem in many larger U.S. teaching hospitals by the early 1980s (Jevons *et al.*, 1963; Panlilio *et al.*, 1992). However, the rapid rise in rates of MRSA in U.S.

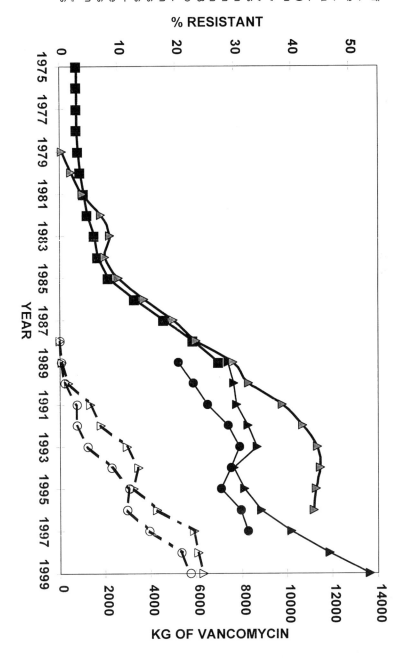

Figure 1. Emergence of MRSA as percentage of *S. aureus* isolates from large teaching hospitals in the U.S. from 1975-1989 (■) and as a percentage of nosocomial *S. aureus* isolates from ICU (▲) and non-ICU (●) settings from 1989-1999. (Panlilio *et al.*, 1992; Fridkin and Gaynes, 1999; Hospital Infections Program, 1999). Also shown are kilograms of vancomycin used worldwide (primarily in the U.S.) from 1979 to 1983 and in the U.S. from 1984 to 1996 (△)(Kirst *et al.*, 1998). The increase in vancomycin consumption closely parallels the increase in MRSA. Rates of VRE in ICU (△) and non-ICU (○) settings begin to rise a decade after the increases in MRSA and vancomycin usage (Fridkin and Gaynes, 1999; Hospital Infections Program, 1999).

hospitals that occurred nationwide in the late 1980's and early 1990's shows no indication of leveling off. In data from the U.S. National Nosocomial Infections Surveillance Program from 1999, MRSA comprised over 50% of intensive care unit *S. aureus* isolates (Hospital Infections Program, 1999). Glycopeptide-resistant strains of enterococci (VRE) arrived more recently than MRSA, but have increased more than 50 fold among isolates from United States hospitals from 1989 to 1999 (Martone, 1998; Murray, 2000).

Resistance has also continued to evolve in other nosocomial gram positive organisms, particularly coagulase negative staphylococci and some streptococci, but the clinical implications of these are less than for *S. aureus* and *Enterococcus*. In this chapter I will discuss pressures leading to the evolution of multi-drug resistant enterococci and staphylococci, their mechanisms of resistance, and implications of the continued spread of these multi-drug resistant pathogens both in and out of the acute hospital setting.

Multidrug Resistant Enterococci and Glycopeptide-Resistant Enterococci

Even prior to the appearance of ampicillin and vancomycin resistance among enterococcal strains, enterococci have assumed increasing importance as hospital pathogens (Schaberg *et al.*, 1991). Enterococci are in many respects ideally suited for the role of nosocomial pathogens. They are hardy organisms that will grow in a wide range of conditions. They colonize the gastrointestinal tract, genitourinary tract and skin of health individuals and persist for long periods of time on environmental surfaces (Murray, 1990; Weber and Rutala, 1997). Even "susceptible" strains of *E. faecalis* and *E. faecium*, the species comprising over 95% of human clinical isolates, are by definition multi-drug resistant. Enterococci are intrinsically resistant to cephalosporins, clindamycin and other lincosamides, and are resistant to aminoglycosides at achievable serum levels. Despite *in vitro* susceptibility, they are also resistant to trimethoprim-sulfamethoxazole *in vivo*. Although susceptible to penicillins, most strains are penicillin tolerant and require much higher penicillin concentrations for inhibition than other streptococci (Tofte *et al.*, 1984; Sherris, 1986).

The overall increase of enterococci as causes of nosocomial bacteremias, urinary tract infections and surgical wound infections is attributed in part to increased use of cephalosporins in the hospital setting (Pallares *et al.*, 1993). Antibiotics active against other normal gastrointestinal flora but not enterococci such as cephalosporins and anti-anaerobic drugs are associated with multi-log increases in fecal enterococcal colony counts, resulting in increased opportunity for infection due to contamination of wounds, intravenous devices and urinary catheters as well as increased risk of endogenous infection from gut translocation (Nord *et al.*, 1984). Increased gastrointestinal shedding of enterococci also promotes contamination of the environment and nosocomial spread on the hands of health care workers (Weber and Rutala, 1997; Donskey *et al.*, 2000). Fortunately, enterococci are not as pathogenic as other gram positives such as *S. aureus* or β-hemolytic streptococci, although several potential virulence factors have recently been identified in *E. faecalis* (Elsner *et al.*, 2000).

Until recently, treatment of enterococcal infections has required either use of a penicillin, generally ampicillin, or vancomycin. These regimens are bacteriostatic against most enterococcal strains. Reliable bactericidal activity, as necessary for treatment of endovascular infections or endocarditis, requires synergistic combinations of a penicillin or glycopeptide with an aminglycoside, most often gentamicin (Calderwood *et al.*, 1977). However, treatment options have been progressively limited by emergence of resistance to all three of these drug classes.

Aminoglycoside Resistance

Low-level aminoglycoside resistance is an intrinsic characteristic of susceptible enterococci. Gentamicin MIC's are commonly 8-32 µg/mL, but aminoglycoside activity is markedly enhanced when combined with a cell wall drug (Calderwood *et al.*, 1977). Nearly all *E. faecium* strains also carry a chromosomal aminotransferase, AAC(6')-Ii, which mediates resistance to tobramycin but not gentamicin (Chow, 2000). High-level gentamicin resistance, mediated predominantly by the bi-functional aminglycoside-inactivating enzyme AAC(6')-APH(2"), first appeared in *E. faecalis* 1978 and has since spread worldwide (Courvalin *et al.*, 1980; Mederski-Samoraj and Murray, 1983; Chow, 2000). Presence of AAC(6')—APH(2") confers resistance to most commercially available aminoglycosides including gentamicin, tobramycin, amikacin, netilmicin and isepamicin (Ferretti *et al.*, 1986).

In most strains aminoglycoside resistance elements are contained on self-transferable plasmids similar to those of staphylococci and streptococci and distinct from those of gram-negative organisms (Chow, 2000). Several additional gentamicin resistance genes of the APH(2")-I class have recently been described in enterococci. One of these, APH2-Ib, has also been found in *E. coli* (Kao *et al.*, 2000). High-level gentamicin resistant enterococci typically have MICs   500 μg/mL and fail to demonstrate any synergy when combined with a cell wall agent. MICs for strains with APH(2")-I genes may be lower. The rapid increase in high-level gentamicin resistant strains during the early 1990's went unnoticed in many hospitals due to the failure of most laboratories to specifically test for this phenotype.

High-level aminoglycoside resistance can be found in up to 50 to 70% of *E. faecalis* isolates in Europe and the U.S. (Schouten *et al.*, 1999; Low *et al.*, 2001). Higher resistance rates are found among nosocomial compared to community strains (Coque *et al.*, 1995). Aminoglycosides are never used alone for treatment of enterococcal infections, thus the primary consequence of this resistance is the inability to achieve bactericidal activity necessary for optimal treatment of endocarditis or endovascular infections. Resistance to streptomycin occurs through different mechanisms, and occasional enterococci may demonstrate β-lactam-streptomycin synergy, although most high-level gentamicin resistant strains also carry streptomycin resistance determinants. In one large study, no significant difference in outcome was demonstrated in patients with *E. faecalis* bacteremia due to high-level gentamicin resistant or non-resistant strains (Watanakunakorn and Patel, 1993).

Penicillin Resistance

Two different mechanisms can result in development of penicillin resistance in enterococci. The first of these, found almost exclusively in *E. faecalis*, is expression of a β-lactamase. First reported in 1983, these penicillin-resistant strains harbor plasmids containing β-lactamases similar to the type A and related β-lactamases of *S. aureus*, but with different mechanisms of regulation and expression (Murray, 1992). β-lactamase and high-level gentamicin resistance genes can be carried on the same conjugative plasmids (Wanger and Murray, 1990). Several nosocomial outbreaks due to strains of β-lactamase producing *E. faecalis* have been described from geographically diverse locations, but such strains are still rare.

The second type of penicillin resistance is mediated by changes in penicillin binding proteins, particularly PBP5. Higher levels of the low penicillin affinity PBP5 or mutations in PBP5 both result in increased penicillin MIC's, although additional mutations may also be required for development of very high-level resistance (Sifaoui *et al.*, 2001). This type of resistance is primarily a characteristic of *E. faecium* and occasionally other species such as *E. raffinosus* (Grayson *et al.*, 1991; Boyce *et al.*, 1992). Most pre-1980's community *E. faecium* strains demonstrated low-level penicillin and ampicillin resistance but by the early 1990's many outbreaks of strains with high-level resistance were being described.

Overall, *E. faecium* have also increased as a proportion of hospital enterococcal isolates (Grayson *et al.*, 1991). Up to 80 to 90% of hospital-acquired *E. faecium* are now ampicillin-resistant with MICs as high as 256-512 µg/mL. Recognition of ampicillin-resistant *E. faecium* as nosocomial pathogens preceded the widespread emergence of vancomycin-resistant *E. faecium*, but the co-evolution of both ampicillin and vancomycin resistance in *E. faecium* has markedly increased the concern about this resistance trait (Handwerger *et al.*, 1992).

Glycopeptide Resistance

Glycopeptide resistant enterococci first appeared in both Europe and the United States in 1986-7, and the first major outbreak was reported from a renal failure unit in England in 1988 (Uttley *et al.*, 1988). Since that time, prevalence of glycopeptide resistant enterococci has continued to increase, although much more so among nosocomial isolates in the United States than other parts of the world, and more in *E. faecium* than any other species (Figure 1, Table 1) (Martone, 1998). Over 90% of hospital VRE isolates are *E. faecium*, the remainder are mostly *E. faecalis*.

Glycopeptide antibiotics are large, bulky heptapeptide molecules that interrupt cell wall synthesis by binding tightly to terminal D-alanyl—D-alanine residues of the cell wall pentapeptide precursor after transport of pentapeptide across the cell membrane, blocking the subsequent

Table 1. Rates of VRE and MRSA in Clinical Isolates from Selected Regions or Countries

Country or Region	MRSA		VRE	
	% Resistant	Time Period (Source)	% Resistant	Time Period (Source)
United States	34	1997-9 (SENTRY)	15	1997-9 (SENTRY)
	21	1995-1997 (TSN)	12	1995-7 (TSN)
	46.5 (ICU) 36 (non-ICU) 21 (outpatient)	1996-2000 (NNIS)	11.3 (ICU) 9.9 (non-ICU) 3.9 (outpatient)	1996-2000 (NNIS)
	29.3	1995-8(SCOPE)	17.7	1995-8 (SCOPE)
Canada	5.7	1997-9 (SENTRY)	1	1997-9 (SENTRY)
Latin America	34.9	1997-9 (SENTRY)	1	1997–9 (SENTRY)
Mexico	11.4	1997-9 (SENTRY)	<1	1997–9 (SENTRY)
Brazil	33.7	1997-9 (SENTRY)	<1	1997–9 (SENTRY)
Denmark	<1	2000 (EARSS)	<1	1997 (EVRE)
Sweden	<1	2000 (EARSS)	0	2001 (EARSS)
The Netherlands	0.5	2000 (EARSS)	0	2001 (EARSS)
Great Britain	39.5	2000 (EARSS)	2.5	1997 (EVRE)

Country				
France	21.4	1997-9 (SENTRY)	<1	1997 (EVRE)
Germany	14.3	2000 (EARSS)	3.8	2000 (EARSS)
Belgium	20.9	2000 (EARSS)	2	2000 (EARSS)
Israel	44.1	2001 (EARSS)	4.6	2001 (EARSS)
Hungary	4	2001 (EARSS)	<1	2001 (EARSS)
Spain	28.1	2000 (EARSS)	0.5	2001 (EARSS)
Greece	38.6	2001(EARSS)	7.8	2001 (EARSS)
Western Pacific	46	1998-9 (SENTRY)	2	1998-9 (SENTRY)
Japan	71.6	1998-9 (SENTRY)	<1	1998-9 (SENTRY)
Australia	23.6	1998-9 (SENTRY)	<1	1998-9 (SENTRY)
Hong Kong	73.8	1998-9 (SENTRY)	<1	1998-9 (SENTRY)

Sources:
SENTRY Antimicrobial Surveillance Program (Diekema et al., 2001; Low et al., 2001)
The Surveillance Network Database (TSN) (Sahm, et al., 1999)
Surveillance and Control of Pathogens of Epidemiologic Importance Database (SCOPE) (Edmond et al., 1999) National Nosocomial Infections Surveillance System (NNIS) (NNIS Semiannual Report, 2001)
European Antimicrobial Resistance Surveillance System (EARSS) (EARSS Database, 2002)
European VRE Study Group (EVRE) (Schouten, et al., 2000)

cell wall synthesis steps of transglycosylation and transpeptidation. The general mechanism of acquired glycopeptide resistance in enterococci involves alteration in the peptidoglycan synthesis pathway so that the pentapeptide D-alanyl—D-alanine terminus is replaced by D-alanyl—D-lactate, or less commonly D-alanyl—D-serine (Fraimow and Courvalin, 2000). Changing the pentapeptide to a D-alanyl—D-lactate terminating depsipeptide eliminates one hydrogen bond in interaction between glycopeptide and the new terminus, resulting in >1000 fold diminished affinity between the glycopeptide and its target (Bugg *et al.*, 1991; Walsh *et al.*, 1996). Several different vancomycin resistance gene clusters have been described (Table 2), but those contributing to the bulk of acquired vancomycin resistance are the *vanA* and *vanB* clusters (Arthur *et al.*, 1996; Fraimow and Courvalin, 2000).

The *vanA* cluster is found predominantly in *E. faecalis* and *E. faecium* but has been reported in most other enterococcal species as well as clinical isolates of *Bacillus*, *Oerskovia* and *Arcanobacterium* (Arthur *et al.*, 1996; Ligozzi *et al.*, 1998). *vanA* has been transferred to other pathogenic gram-positives in the laboratory, including *Listeria* and *S. aureus* (Noble *et al.*, 1992). The *vanA* gene has also recently been found in a clinical methicillin-resistant *S. aureus* isolate demonstrating high level vancomycin resistance (CDC, 2002). VanA type resistance is usually but not invariably plasmid-mediated, most commonly as part of the transposon Tn*1546* (Arthur *et al.*, 1993).

Essential genes of the *vanA* cluster include the *vanA* gene encoding a D-alanyl—D-lactate ligase for synthesis of the D-alanyl—D-lactate moiety; *vanH* encoding a lactate dehydrogenase for the synthesis of D-lactate, and *vanX* encoding a D-D dipeptidase required to eliminate D-alanyl—D-alanine synthesized through the normal cell wall synthetic pathway. The other essential genes of the *vanA* cluster encode for VanRS. VanRS is a two-component regulator that directly or indirectly senses vancomycin and up-regulates expression of the other essential genes (Arthur *et al.*, 1992).

Induction of the *vanA* cluster also occurs following exposure to bacitracin and the transglycosylase inhibitor moenomycin, suggesting that the signal for induction is an indirect effect of vancomycin exposure rather than vancomycin (Arthur and Quintiliani, 2001). Other genes of the cluster include *vanY* which encodes for a carboxypeptidase and *vanZ*, an auxiliary gene of unknown function. Tn*1546* also contains transposase and resolvase genes. Induction of expression of the *vanA*

Table 2. Genotypic and phenotypic characterization of Glycopeptide resistant enterococci

Resistance Genotype	Predominant Phenotype*	Mode of Expression	Predominant Location	Transferable Elements	Alternate Precursor	Species Found in
vanA	Va ≥ 256 T Te ≥ 32	inducible	Plasmid (chromosome**)	Tn1546 and related	D-Ala–D-Lac	E. faecium, E.faecalis, E.avium, E.durans E.mundtii, E.hirae***, O. turbata, B.circulans A.haemolyticum, S.aureus
vanB	Va 4 to1000 Te 1	inducible	Chromosome (plasmid**)	eg. Tn1547 Tn5382	D-Ala–D-Lac	E. faecium, E.faecalis. S. bovis
vanC1 vanC2 vanC3	Va 2 to 32 Te 1	constitutive or inducible	Chromosome	none?	D-Ala–D-Ser	E.gallinarum (vanC1) E.casseliflavus(vanC2) E. flavescens (vanC3)
vanD1-4	Va 64 to 256 Te 4 to 32	constitutive or inducible	Chromosome	?	D-Ala–D-Lac	E. faecium
vanE	Va = 16 Te = 0.5	inducible	Chromosome?	?	D-Ala–D-Ser	E. faecalis
vanG	Va = 16 Te = 0.5	?	Chromosome?	?	D-Ala–D-Ser?	E. faecalis

* Expressed as MIC to Vancomycin (Va) or Teicoplanin (Te) in μg/ml   ** rare isolates described   *** and other enterococcal species
Data for vanE and vanG are based on a single isolate or cluster

cluster causes high-level resistance to both vancomycin (MIC 256 µg/mL) and teicoplanin (MIC 32 µg/mL).

The *vanB* system is structurally similar to the *vanA* cluster, consisting of the D-alanyl—D-lactate ligase gene *vanB* as well as dehydrogenase and dipeptidase genes, all of which have 65-75% amino-acid identity with their *vanA* counterparts (Arthur *et al.*, 1996). VanB also contains a two-component regulator VanR$_B$S$_B$ functionally similar but genetically distinct from the VanRS system with only 34 and 23% amino acid identity with *vanR* and *vanS* (Evers and Courvalin, 1996). The *vanB* cluster also contains a *vanY*-like carboxypeptidase and a novel gene, *vanW*, of unknown function. Several slightly different variants of *vanB* have been described (Gold *et al.*, 1993).

The *vanB* cluster is found almost exclusively in *E. faecium* and *E. faecalis* and results in variable levels of vancomycin resistance with MICs of 4 to >1000 µg/mL. Unlike *vanA* strains, *vanB* strains are typically susceptible teicoplanin due to failure of teicoplanin to induce expression of the *vanB* cluster via the VanS$_B$ sensor. Teicoplanin resistance can develop from constitutive expression of *vanB* or specific mutations in *vanS$_B$* that change specificity of the glycopeptide sensor (Arthur and Quintiliani, 2001). Initial studies indicated that *vanB* was found in the chromosome on large transposable elements such as Tn*1547* and Tn*5382*, but more recently plasmids containing the *vanB* cluster have also been described (Rice *et al.*, 1998). In some strains the Tn*5382* *vanB* resistance cluster is physically associated with a *pbp5* sequence that co-transfers with *vanB* as part of a larger mobile element, facilitating dissemination of both vancomycin and high-level ampicillin resistance between *E. faecium* strains (Carias *et al.*, 1998).

The *vanC* clusters are intrinsic to the less clinically important, motile enterococcal species *E. casseliflavus*, *E. flavescens* and *E. gallinarum* and result in either constitutive or inducible low level vancomycin resistance by producing the dipeptide D-alanyl—D-serine rather than D-alanyl—D-alanine as their pentapeptide terminus (Navarro and Courvalin, 1994; Arias *et al.*, 2000). Other acquired vancomycin resistance clusters that have been reported in small numbers of *E. faecium* or *E. faecalis* isolates include the *vanD*, *vanE* and *vanG* clusters.

The several variants of the *vanD* cluster are structurally similar to *vanA* and are also mediated through production of a D-alanyl—D-lactate terminating alternate precursor and demonstrate intermediate to high-level glycopeptide resistance (Casadewall and Courvalin, 1999). The *vanE* and the *vanG* clusters are most similar to *vanC* systems in that resistance is mediated through production of D-alanyl—D-serine resulting in a low level vancomycin resistance (Fines *et al.*, 1999; McKessar *et al.*, 2000). Genotyping of VRE strains for identification of specific resistance genes is not routinely performed in clinical laboratories and phenotypic methods are unreliable in distinguishing between different genotypes, thus there may be additional resistance clusters present among clinical isolates that have not yet been characterized.

The origins of *vanA*, *vanB* and other acquired vancomycin resistance clusters is unknown but their complex structure, location on transposons and differences in G+C content from the remainder of the enterococcal genome strongly suggest origins in other species (Arthur *et al.*, 1996). The mechanism of acquired enterococcal resistance is different than that in intrinsically glycopeptide-resistant lactic acid producing gram-positives such as *Pediococcus*, *Leuconostoc* and *Lactobacillus*. These also produce depsipeptide terminating in D-alanyl—D-lactate rather than D-alanyl—D-alanine, but the ligases in these organisms are of distinct genetic lineage from *vanA* and *vanB* (Evers *et al.*, 1996). Glycopeptide producing organisms are natural candidates for production of glycopeptide resistance genes. The glycopeptide producing *Streptomyces toyocaensis* and *Amycolaptis orientalis* contain clusters consisting of a lactate dehydrogenase, D-alanyl—D-lactate ligase and D-D dipeptidase with 50-65% amino acid homology with *vanHAX* and *vanH$_B$BX$_B$* but with G+C content much closer to that of the G+C rich *Actinomycetes* (Marshall *et al.*, 1997; Marshall *et al.*, 1998).

One attractive hypothesis is that glycopeptide resistance genes may have been acquired from *Streptomyces* species by bacilli or other non-pathogenic environmental gram-positives that have capability for direct gene transfer to enterococci. Support for this comes from the recent finding of a glycopeptide resistance cluster with 70-75% homology to the *vanA* cluster located on a probable transposon in environmental isolates of the soil-dwelling biopesticide *Paenibacillus popilliae* (Patel *et al.*, 2000). In one resistant *P. popilliae* strain, a short nucleotide sequence identical to a portion of the transposase gene of the *vanA* Tn*1546* transposon is found adjacent to the glycopeptide resistance cluster (H.S. Fraimow, unpublished).

Epidemiology of Vancomycin Resistant Enterococci (VRE)

The epidemiology of glycopeptide or vancomycin resistant enterococci (generally referred to as VRE) is quite different in Europe and the U.S., providing some insight into the selective pressures necessary for emergence and persistence of these strains (Table 1). Although VRE remain quite rare in healthy individuals without hospital exposures in the U.S., rates of nosocomial VRE are much higher than in Europe (Goossens, 1998). Rising rates of VRE in U.S. hospitals temporally follow the upswing in vancomycin use that occurred during the late 1980s and 1990s in response to the increasing prevalence of MRSA (Figure 1) (Kirst *et al.*, 1998). It is thus reasonable to propose that the primary initial selective pressure for emergence of VRE in the U.S has been hospital vancomycin usage.

In Europe, VRE can be isolated at moderate frequency from stool of healthy volunteers, although hospital rates remain low (Van der Auwera *et al.*, 1996). There is also significant genetic diversity among community isolates, suggesting that selective pressure for emergence of VRE has occurred at multiple locations outside of the hospital. VRE have also been isolated from other environmental sources including raw sewage, animal carcasses and ground meat, suggesting routes of spread throughout the human food chain (Klare *et al.*, 1993; Goossens, 1998).

Speculation has focused on role of avoparcin, a glycopeptide antibiotic approved for use in several European countries as a feed additive in the 1970's but never approved for use in the U.S. Rates of VRE have generally been higher in European countries where avoparcin has been used. Within countries, poultry and pig farms using avoparcin had much higher rates of recovery of VRE than antibiotic-free farms (Aarestrup, 1995). Faced with this epidemiologic data, many European countries banned the use of avoparcin as well as other antimicrobial agents as growth promoters. In one recent study from Denmark, rates of vancomycin resistant *E. faecium* in broiler chickens fell from 73% in 1995, the year of the avoparcin ban, to 5.8% by 2000 (Aarestrup *et al.*, 2001).

Concern regarding use of antibiotics animal feed supplements has expanded beyond glycopeptides to other agent that may either co-select for vancomycin and multi-drug resistance or that may have clinical relevance for treatment of human enterococcal infections. Unlike rates in poultry farms, rates of VRE in pig farms in Denmark did not immediately decrease after elimination of avoparcin use. Ongoing use of the macrolide tylosin in pig farms may have resulted in continuing co-selection for both glycopeptide and macrolide resistance in *E. faecium* strains (Aarestrup *et al.*, 2001). One example of an agriculturally important agent that may have implications for treatment of human infections is virginiamycin, a combination streptogramin very similar to quinupristin-dalfopristin, an agent recently approved for treatment of VRE faecium. Usage of virginiamycin has now been linked to recovery of quinupristin-dalfopristin resistant enterococci from poultry flocks as well as from broiler chickens sold at supermarkets in the U.S. (McDonald *et al.*, 2001).

Epidemiology of VRE in the Hospital Environment

Rates of VRE in U.S. hospitals have increased yearly since 1989 (Figure 1) (Martone, 1998; Fridkin and Gaynes, 1999; Murray, 2000). In the U.S., the hospital environment remains the reservoir for most VRE infections. Numerous studies have addressed the nosocomial epidemiology of VRE. Some patient-specific risk factors for colonization or infection with VRE that have been identified repeatedly in multi-variant analyses include prolonged hospital stay, intensive care unit exposure, hematologic malignancies, transplantation, gastrointestinal manipulations and enteral feeding (Morris *et al.*, 1995; Tornieporth *et al.*, 1996; Bonten *et al.*, 1998; Martone, 1998).

In all studies, however, the single most important risk factor for increased risk of VRE for both individual patients and among institutions has been antibiotic exposure. Not surprisingly, the strongest association is with either parenteral or oral vancomycin usage. In other studies exposure to 3rd generation cephalosporins and to anti-anaerobic drugs including metronidazole and clindamycin is also implicated (Martone, 1998; Rice, 2001). The "intensity" of antibiotic exposure (number and duration of antibiotics) has also been associated with VRE acquisition (Morris *et al.*, 1995; Tornieporth *et al.*, 1996; Bonten *et al.*, 1998). Antibiotic pressure may act in several ways to increase the spread of

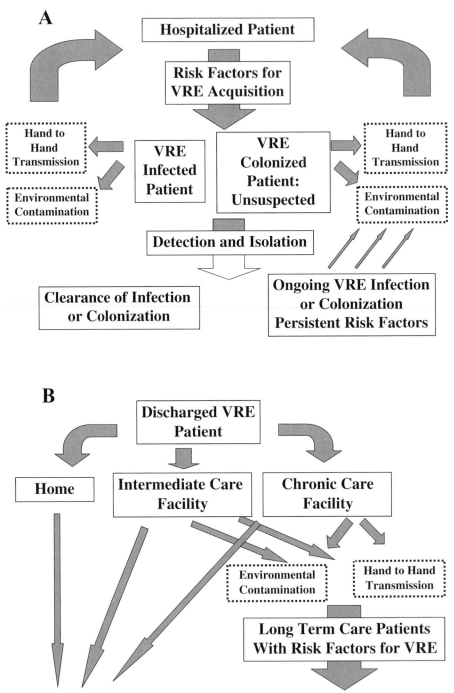

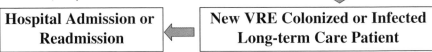

Figure 2. Flow of VRE and VRE infected or colonized patients through the healthcare system. **(A)** Hospitalized patients exposed to VRE with risk factors for VRE acquisition (see text) become colonized or infected with VRE. These unrecognized VRE patients shed VRE into their environment, predominantly from the GI tract, leading to nosocomial transmission on the hands of health care personnel. Once they are identified and appropriately isolated, some patients will clear their VRE, but most will remain colonized and pose a decreased but ongoing risk for transmission. **(B)** Colonized patients may be discharged home; or may go to intermediate or chronic care facilities, resulting in further transmission to other at risk patients. Patients with persistent VRE as well as their now colonized contacts may then be readmitted to acute care hospitals, perpetuating the cycle of transmission. Similar processes are also important in the transmission of other nosocomial resistant pathogens.

VRE in the hospital setting (Figure 2). In non-colonized patients newly admitted to the hospital, exposure to antibiotics active against normal fecal flora but not enterococci provides a greater opportunity for establishment of persistent colonization by VRE. In *in vitro* and animal models, antibiotics promote establishment of VRE colonization but "healthy" human fecal flora is resistant to VRE colonization (Donskey *et al.*, 2000; 2001).

Once a patient becomes colonized with VRE through person to person transmission or environmental contamination, ongoing exposure to antibiotics not active against VRE (*e.g.*, vancomycin) as well as those active against other components of the upper and lower gastrointestinal flora (*e.g.*, 3rd generation cephalosporins, clindamycin, metronidazole) can contribute to expansion of the fecal enterococcal population (Donskey *et al.*, 2000). Higher fecal VRE concentrations are associated with higher risk of environmental contamination and secondary spread.

Persistence of VRE in the hospital is facilitated by large numbers of "silent" carriers with fecal colonization, who may outnumber infected patients by more than 5 to 1 (Figure 2) (Bonten *et al.*, 1998). Screening for VRE colonization with selective media can detect as few as 10^3 cfu of VRE of per gram of stool, but patients initially colonized with even fewer organisms may subsequently shed VRE at high numbers following antibiotic exposures. Diarrhea and fecal incontinence also contribute to increased environmental contamination and higher skin colonization rates (Boyce *et al.*, 1994b). Once fecal colonization occurs, it can persist for up to 1 to 2 years even after elimination of antibiotic selective pressure (Lai *et al.*, 1997). Hospital units where patients require prolonged hospitalization and frequent readmission, high intensity antibiotic exposure and high use of invasive devices would be predicted to have ongoing problems with VRE. Hematology-oncology units and liver transplant units are foci of many of the ongoing VRE outbreaks that have been reported.

Table 3. Strategies for Preventing Transmission of MRSA and VRE in Health Care Facilities

Strategy	For VRE?	For MRSA?
Control of Antimicrobial Usage		
Restrict all unnecessary antimicrobial therapy	++	++
Restriction of specific drugs and duration of Rx for surgical prophylaxis	++*	++
Restriction of specific classes of antimicrobials		
Vancomycin (oral and IV)	++*	?
3rd Generation Cephalosporins	+	?
Anti-anaerobic drugs	?	?
Educational Programs		
On antibiotic prescribing (for physicians)	++	++
On transmission of resistant organisms (for all health care providers)	++*	++
Microbiology Testing Procedures		
Optimize methods for detecting resistance in significant clinical isolates	++*	++
Testing of resistant isolates against appropriate alternative drugs	++*	++
Periodic susceptibility testing of non-significant isolates	++*	++
Processing of surveillance cultures	++	++
Use of molecular strain typing methods	+ outbreaks only	+ outbreaks only
Use of Isolation and Barrier Precautions		
Handwashing with soap and water or antimicrobial soap, alcohol gels	++*	++
Gloves required for all patient contact	++*	+ (? NP)
Gloves required for dressing changes and wound care	++	++
Gowns for all patient contact	+	?
Gowns for patient and environment contact where soiling is expected	++*	++
Dedicated stethoscopes and personal care equipment	++*	?
Private rooms or cohorting	++*	+ (? NP)
Isolation wards if prevalence rates high	+*	+
Dedicated staff for colonized or infected patients if rates high	+*	+

Housekeeping Measures

Cleaning/ disinfecting of patient areas after discharge or transfer	++*	++
Cleaning/ disinfection of reusable equipment	++*	++

Surveillance Activities

Routine review of susceptibility data from microbiology laboratory	++*	++
Routine surveillance cultures in low incidence areas	+*	?
Routine surveillance cultures in high incidence areas	+	+
Surveillance cultures on transfer from high to low incidence areas	+	+
Surveillance of contacts/roommates of newly identified cases	+*	?
Flagging of colonized patients for identification on transfer/readmission	++*	++
Surveillance cultures to determine when patients are no longer colonized	++* rectal, other	+ NP, skin, other
Surveillance cultures of health care personnel	?	+ outbreaks

Decontamination of Colonized with Antimicrobial Agents

Topical decontamination of nasopharynx (NP)	?	+
Gastrointestinal decontamination	?	?
Topical decontamination of skin sites/open wounds	?	?
Systemic antimicrobial agents	?	?
Decontamination of colonized health care workers	?	+ outbreaks

*	Components of HICPAC Recommendations for Preventing Spread of Vancomycin Resistance (H.I.C.P.A.C., 1995)
++	Applicable in most circumstances; recommended by most expert panels
+	Applicable or recommended in only specific circumstances; or recommended by only some expert panels
?	Data incomplete or inconclusive
?	No evidence to support this, not recommended
?NP	May not be applicable to patients with only nasopharyngeal colonization

Changes in healthcare practices over the past decade have further complicated the epidemiology of VRE in the U.S. Acute hospitalizations are shorter and many patients are subsequently transferred to intermediate care nursing facilities, rehabilitation facilities and nursing homes for completion of treatment, which often includes parenteral antibiotic therapy. Thus colonized patients can continue to shed VRE surrounded by other debilitated, at-risk patients in institutions where infection control practices may be less rigorous than those in acute care hospitals. Readmission of unsuspected VRE colonized patients from chronic care centers back to the acute care setting provides further opportunity for unsuspected hospital environmental contamination and ongoing transmission (Figure 2).

Strategies for Control of VRE

Control of VRE involves cohesive efforts on behalf of clinicians, clinical microbiologists, pharmacists, hospital epidemiologists and infection control practitioners and hospital administrators. Specific recommendations designed to control the spread of VRE have been made by the U.S. Hospital Infection Control Practices Advisory Committee (Table 3) (H.I.C.P.A.C., 1995). These recommendations were initially formulated in response to rising VRE rates without proof of their effectiveness, but there is now increasing evidence that implementation can be useful for control of new VRE outbreaks with limited numbers of infected and colonized patients (Ostrowsky *et al.*, 2001). However, it is less certain that they will be effective for long-term VRE outbreaks in institutions with high VRE prevalence, large reservoirs of colonized patients and ongoing selective pressure from both glycopeptide and non-glycopeptide antibiotic use (Morris *et al.*, 1995; Lai *et al.*, 1998). High "colonization pressure", defined as the proportion of patients in a unit already colonized with VRE, may result in failure to eliminate VRE despite adherence to HICPAC guidelines (Bonten *et al.*, 1998).

Imposition of strict criteria for vancomycin usage can significantly reduce glycopeptide consumption, though such reductions may be more difficult in institutions with very high rates of MRSA. Restricting other antibiotics in addition to vancomycin may be necessary for control of VRE. Several studies suggest that 3rd generation cephalosporin but not piperacillin or piperacillin-tazobactam exposure may be associated with increased VRE rates, and that modifications of patterns of broad-spectrum antibiotic usage through formulary restrictions may be helpful in control of VRE (Quale *et al.*, 1996; Donskey *et al.*, 2000; Fridkin *et al.*, 2001; Rice, 2001). Elimination of any unnecessary antibiotic exposure is an appropriate goal for all institutions.

Treatment with oral, non-absorbable antibiotics is a theoretically attractive approach for selective gut decolonization by VRE. However, there are few available agents that are active against multidrug-resistant enterococci that do not also have some potential role for treatment of systemic VRE infections. In small trials, bacitracin demonstrated only transient decrease in fecal colonization levels when used alone or in combination therapy (Weinstein *et al.*, 1999). In a trial of ramoplanin, an experimental, non-absorbable glycolipodepsipeptide active against VRE, there was also transient but not sustained clearing of VRE (Wong *et al.*, 2001). However, even transient decolonization may be beneficial in defined populations at periods of high risk, such as neutropenic patients or patients undergoing liver transplantation.

Consequences of VRE Infection and Treatment of VRE

There have been numerous descriptions of serious morbidity and mortality associated with VRE infections, especially bacteremia and endovascular infections. However, it has been more difficult to prove that vancomycin resistance and the associated delay in appropriate therapy is an independent determinant of mortality from enterococcal infection. Many episodes of enterococcal bacteremia are self-limited or respond to removal of infected lines or devices without effective antimicrobial therapy. A recent study prospectively analyzed 398 episodes of enterococcal bacteremia and did confirm vancomycin resistance to be an independent predictor of mortality, and that earlier initiation of appropriate therapy resulted in improved survival (Vergis *et al.*, 2001).

Treatment of VRE has been limited by lack of effective agents for these usually multi-resistant infections (Table 4). Over 99% of vancomycin-resistant *E. faecalis* strains remain susceptible to penicillins, thus treatment of these is problematic primarily in penicillin allergic patients or those requiring bactericidal therapy. Those rare infections due to vancomycin-resistant β-lactamase producing *E. faecalis* can be treated with β-lactamase inhibitor combination drugs such as ampicillin-sulbactam. Treatment of vancomycin-resistant *E. faecium* (VREF) poses a much greater challenge. Most VREF have ampicillin MICs >64 μg/mL,

Table 4. Resistance of VRE and MRSA in the U.S. to Other Antimicrobial Agents, 1997-1999

Susceptibility of MRSA 34% of *S. aureus* Isolates		Susceptibility of VRE 15% of Enterococcal Isolates*	
Antimicrobial	**% Susceptible**	**Antimicrobial**	**% Susceptible**
Trimethoprim-sulfamethoxazole	74	Ampicillin	96 (*E. faecalis*)
Rifampin	90		1 (*E. faecium*)
Gentamicin	63	Gentamicin-HL	40
Clindamycin	20	Streptomycin-HL	21
Erythromycin	6	Erythromycin	3
Chloramphenicol	52	Chloramphenicol	90
Tetracycline	90	Doxycycline	53
Ciprofloxacin	10	Ciprofloxacin	3
Vancomycin	100**	Nitrofurantoin	40
Quinupristin-Dalfopristin	98	Quinupristin-Dalfpristin	96 (*E. faecium* only)
Linezolid	100***	Linezolid	100***

 * Species are not specified for all strains in SENTRY database, but from other studies > 80% of VRE are *E. faecium* and ~ 50% of *E. faecium* are vancomycin-resistant; 10 to 20% of VRE are *E. faecalis* and 2 to 3% of *E. faecalis* are vancomycin-resistant (Edmond *et al.*, 1999: Sahm *et al.*, 1999) ** But 0.3% have MIC =4 µg/ml; several reports of strains with MIC $\geq$ 8 µg/ml *** Reports of intermediately susceptible or fully resistant strains. From: SENTRY Antimicrobial Surveillance Program (Diekema *et al.*, 2001; Low *et al.*, 2001).

above levels achievable even with high dose therapy. Until recently, initial therapy for such VREF strains relied either on older, bacteriostatic drugs or combinations of several agents that might demonstrate additive effects *in vitro* (Murray, 2000). Many strains of VREF have been susceptible *in vitro* to tetracyclines and chloramphenicol. Doxycycline and chloramphenicol have both been used extensively for treatment of VREF with evidence of clinical response, though benefits on survival are less clear-cut (Lautenbach *et al.*, 1998; Murray, 2000). Unfortunately, tetracycline resistance mediated by either efflux pumps (such as TetK or L) or by ribosomal protection (such as TetM, O, S or U) has become more prevalent among *E. faecium* over the past decade. Only 50% of VRE were susceptible to doxycyline in one recent survey (Low *et al.*,

2001). Minocycline may be active against some tetracycline resistant strains. Prevalence of chloramphenicol resistance, mediated by CAT enzymes, remains low in the U.S. Although most enterococci were susceptible to the fluoroquinolone ciprofloxacin when this drug was initially introduced, high-level fluoroquinolone resistance has emerged rapidly due to the selection of topoisomerase and gyrase mutants (Brisse *et al.*, 1999).

Newer quinolones with enhanced gram-positive activity such as clinafloxacin, moxifloxacin and gemifloxacin are intrinsically more active against enterococci, but not against strains that are already ciprofloxacin resistant, and show inconsistent effects in animal models (Brisse *et al.*, 1999; Murray, 2000). They should not be used as monotherapy for treatment of life-threatening enterococcal infection. Macrolide resistance determinants, including novel efflux pumps and *erm* methylases, are also widely distributed in enterococci (Portillo *et al.*, 2000). Rifampin remains active against many resistant enterococcal strains but is only bacteriostatic and cannot be used alone due rapid emergence of resistance. The contribution of rifampin to multi-drug combination regimens remains unclear. Multi-drug combinations of weakly active or inactive drugs such as ampicillin + vancomycin + gentamicin have been extensively studied in *in vitro* and animal models and may be bactericidal against individual strains, but no single combination demonstrates efficacy against a broad range of clinical VREF isolates (Fraimow and Venuti, 1992).

One positive consequence of emergence of VREF and other gram-positive multi-resistant superbugs has been to revitalize the area of gram-positive antimicrobial drug development. The U.S. Food and Drug Administration recently approved two novel agents partly on the basis of their activity against VREF. Quinupristin-dalfopristin (Synercid) is a parenteral combination antibiotic composed of streptogramin A and B components with synergistic activity against different targets in the bacterial 50S ribosome (Moellering *et al.*, 1999). Quinupristin-dalfopristin is active against *E. faecium* but not *E. faecalis* strains and has been effective against VRE infection in clinical trails and in compassionate use programs (Moellering *et al.*, 1999). Linezolid (Zyvox) is the first of the oxazolidinones, a novel class of agents that target a later step in protein synthesis. First approved for use in 2000, linezolid demonstrates potent but bacteriostatic activity against *E. faecium* and *E. faecalis* and other resistant gram-positive pathogens, and offers the advantage of bioequivalence of the oral and parenteral formulations (Diekema and Jones, 2001).

Resistance to both these agents was quite rare in initial susceptibility surveys and difficult to select for *in vitro*. Not surprisingly, however, resistance to both quinupristin-dalfopristin and linezolid has emerged during treatment of VREF infections. 4% of patients treated in the quinupristin-dalfopristin emergency-use program had emergence of resistance on therapy (Linden *et al.*, 2001). Resistance determinants for either streptogramin A or streptogramin B have been found in clinical VREF isolates as well as agricultural isolates, especially from farms where virginiamycin has been used. In recent data from the SENTRY Antimicrobial Surveillance Program, 3.8% of *E. faecium* clinical isolates were quinupristin-dalfopristin resistant, and in Germany up to 14% of healthy adults carry resistant *E. faecium* strains in their stool (Werner *et al.*, 2000; Low *et al.*, 2001).

One environmental *E. faecium* isolate contained both streptogramin A and B resistance determinants in a single transposon (Jensen *et al.*, 2000). Resistance to linezolid *in vitro* results from sequential accumulation of mutations in several copies of the peptidyl transferase region of the multi-copy 23S ribosomal RNA sequence, and resistance has now been found in clinical *E. faecium* isolates (Gonzales *et al.*, 2001; Prystowsky *et al.*, 2001). With increased use of these new agents, resistance will likely increase through nosocomial dissemination of quinupristin-dalfopristin or linezolid resistant VREF as well as through ongoing selection of resistant strains from patients on therapy who have high organism burdens or difficult to eradicate sites of infection. Usage of these drugs must be carefully controlled to try and preserve their effectiveness.

Even as resistance is emerging to these newest agents, other novel antimicrobial agents active against VREF are progressing in clinical trials. These include LY33328, a modified glycopeptide agent with enhanced potency and a novel mechanism of action against VRE; everninomycin, an oligosaccharide agent; and glycylcycline tetracycline derivatives. Daptomycin, a lipopeptide compound initially studied for gram positive infections over a decade ago, has been redeveloped and used successfully for treatment of VREF infections in clinical trials and is currently under FDA review (Tally and DeBruin, 2000). Unfortunately, resistance to all of these agents has already been seen *in vitro* or in animal isolates and thus would be predicted to emerge *in vivo*. Judicious use of all these newer agents will be critical for prolonging their "window of usefulness" for treatment of VREF.

Methicillin Resistant *Staphylococcus aureus*

Staphylococcus aureus continues to be the single most important cause of nosocomial infections from all sites, and is the most common pathogen identified in nosocomial bacteremias, wound infections and pneumonias in the U.S. (Hospital Infections Program, National Center for Infectious Diseases, 1999). *S. aureus* has followed a different pathway of evolution into a multidrug resistant pathogen than *Enterococcus*. Unlike the more intrinsically resistant but less virulent enterococcus, preantibiotic-era staphylococci were exquisitely susceptible to the antibiotics developed in the 1940's and 1950's. When first introduced, penicillin was highly effective against almost all *S. aureus* strains (Plorde and Sherris, 1974).

The emergence of plasmid-mediated β-lactamase production and rapid dissemination of these plasmids in nosocomial *S. aureus* and coagulase negative staphylococci during the 1950's markedly limited the usefulness of penicillin for staphylococcal infections. By 1980, over 80% of both nosocomial and community *S. aureus* isolates were penicillin resistant (Chambers, 2001). Despite their widespread geographic dissemination, only a limited array of staphylococcal β-lactamase genes have been identified (Voladri *et al.*, 1996). These primarily plasmid mediated β-lactamases and associated regulatory genes are often incorporated into transposons such as Tn*552*, Tn*4002* and Tn*4201*. In many early penicillin-resistant strains, β-lactamase genes were associated with genes encoding resistance to mercury and other heavy metals and disinfectants (Lyon and Skurray, 1987).

The rapid dissemination of β-lactamase producing *S. aureus* suggests that factors other than human penicillin exposure have contributed to their emergence. β-lactamase producing *S. aureus* are found among strains predating the clinical use of penicillin (Lyon and Skurray, 1987). By the end of the 1950's many hospital strains had also acquired resistance to the other available antimicrobials including erythromycin, tetracycline and streptomycin (Plorde and Sherris, 1974). The β-lactamase stable semi-synthetic penicillins methicillin, nafcillin and oxacillin were first introduced in 1959 to combat penicillin-resistant staphylococci, but by 1960 the first methicillin-resistant *S. aureus* strains already appeared in England (Jevons *et al.*, 1963). Although methicillin is no longer used either clinically or for *in vitro* susceptibility testing, the name methicillin-resistant *S. aureus* (MRSA) remains deeply entrenched in the literature, although some authors use the more clinically relevant term "oxacillin-resistant".

Mechanism of Resistance in MRSA

Staphylococcal resistance to the semi-synthetic penicillins, also referred to as "intrinsic" resistance, is mediated through changes in PBPs. This can occur either through acquisition of novel PBPs or less commonly by modification in one of the four preexisting staphylococcal PBPs (Chambers, 1997). In most instances resistance is due to the presence of the *mec* gene cluster and results in production of penicillin binding protein PBP2a in addition to the other staphylococcal PBPs (Hartman and Tomasz, 1984). The *mecA* gene encoding for PBP2a is contained in a larger cluster of 30-60 kb of DNA incorporated into restricted sites in the staphylococcal chromosome (Archer and Niemeyer, 1994; Chambers, 2001). The *mec* cluster also includes the *mecI* and *mecR1* genes that regulate expression of *mecA*, in addition to variable amounts of additional DNA.

This additional DNA can include genes encoding for resistance to heavy metals, erythromycin, tetracycline or aminoglycosides, a variety of insertional sequences, and recombinases for mobilization of the *mec* element (Chambers, 2001). There are four types of *mec* resistance determinants, each with a unique pattern of associated genetic material. When present, PBP2a becomes the primary transpeptidase in staphylococcal cell wall synthesis. The currently available β-lactam agents bind less avidly to PBP2a than to other staphylococcal PBPs, resulting in lack of inhibition of cell wall synthesis. Binding of some agents is more dramatically affected *in vitro* than others, resulting in inconsistent *in vitro* susceptibility testing using different β-lactams (Chambers *et al.*, 1990).

Expression of *mecA* can be either constitutive or inducible depending on associated regulatory elements. Constitutive expression results in a homogenously resistant phenotype, inducible expression results in a hetero-resistant phenotype. The degree of expression can vary greatly depending on many environmental factors. Multiple other chromosomal genes in the cell wall biosynthesis and autolysis pathways such as *fem* genes affect expression of resistance (de Lencastre and Tomasz, 1994). The staphylococcal β-lactamase regulatory genes *blaI* and *blaR1* are homologous with the *mecA* regulatory genes *mecI* and *mecR1*, and are also important for control of *mecA* (Chambers, 1997).

Other mechanisms besides PBP2a production can also be associated with low levels of methicillin resistance. *In vitro*, mutations in PBP2 and alteration of expression of PBP4 are each associated with increased methicillin MICs in *mecA* negative strains (Berger-Bachi *et al.*, 1986). Hyper-production of β-lactamase, usually found in association with PBP changes, may also contribute to low-level methicillin resistance (McDougal and Thornsberry, 1986). Using genotypic methods for detection of *mecA*, it is apparent that these rare *mecA* negative, methicillin-resistant clinical isolates express only low-level resistance (Chambers, 1997). They are primarily important in that they are difficult to distinguish in the laboratory from some hetero-resistant *mecA* strains. In addition to true resistance to semi-synthetic penicillins, another characteristic of uncertain clinical significance in some *S. aureus* strains is the phenomenon of "tolerance", or loss of bactericidal activity of β-lactam drugs (Handwerger and Tomasz, 1985).

Recent genetic studies of the insertional sites and sequences of *mec* elements in geographically diverse MRSA strains suggest that acquisition of *mecA* by *S. aureus* resulted from a limited number of unique insertional events into the genome of susceptible *S. aureus*, followed by global dissemination of these MRSA clones (Kreiswirth *et al.*, 1993). *mecA* genes are also highly conserved in other species of staphylococci. The origin of the *mecA* cluster is unknown but is likely to have evolved from another, non-pathogenic staphylococcus species such as *Staphylococcus scuiri* or similar species. Nearly all *S. scuiri* strains contain a *mecA*-like gene with 88% amino-acid homology to *mecA*, but do not express a methicillin-resistant phenotype (Wu *et al.*, 2001). Insertion of this gene into *mecA*-negative *S. aureus* results in expression of methicillin resistance.

Epidemiology of MRSA

The first reported hospital outbreaks of MRSA occurred in the mid 1960's in Europe (Parker and Hewitt, 1970). By the late 1960's outbreaks were also being reported from the U.S. (Barrett *et al.*, 1968). The National

Nosocomial Infectious Surveillance System has tracked the rate of nosocomial MRSA infections in a cohort of U.S. hospitals of since 1975 (Figure 1) (Panlilio et al., 1992). Rates of MRSA began to rise dramatically in large university teaching hospitals in the early 1980's, followed by increases in smaller community hospitals. By 1991, 97% of hospitals were reporting the presence of MRSA strains. Despite recognition of the problem and implementation of guidelines for control of MRSA in most hospitals, overall rates of nosocomial MRSA continue to increase annually (Figure 1). By 1999, 54.5% of ICU *S. aureus* isolates in the U.S. were methicillin resistant, an increase of 43% from the rate in 1994-1998 (Hospital Infections Program, 1999). Globally, MRSA have also become established worldwide, though rates vary markedly in different countries (Table 1). For example, in Europe in 1991, rates ranged from less than 1% in Denmark to over 30% in France and Italy (Voss et al., 1994). However, even regions with traditionally lower rates of MRSA such as Scandinavia still experience periodic outbreaks.

Within the hospital environment, multiple risk factors for colonization and subsequent infection with MRSA have been repeatedly described (Boyce et al., 1994a; Herwaldt, 1999). These include prolonged hospital stay, intensive care unit or burn unit stay, surgical wounds, chronic underlying diseases such as renal failure and malignancy, and prolonged exposure to antimicrobial agents, especially broad spectrum agents. In patients without MRSA on entry to the hospital, initial colonization most likely occurs via transient carriage of organisms by health care workers from colonized or infected patient or less commonly from chronically colonized health care workers (Sheretz et al., 1996; Boyce, 2001). MRSA can persist on environmental surfaces for varying periods of time, and environmental contamination may also be important, particularly from colonized patients with large organism burdens (Boyce et al., 1997).

Colonization can initially occur at a variety of sites, including open wounds, the respiratory tract (especially in ventilator-dependent or tracheostomy patients), around indwelling lines or devices, and in the perineal area, as well as on intact skin and in the nasopharynx (Boyce, 2001). Some sites, such as large open wounds and the respiratory tract of tracheostomy patients, are more important reservoirs of secondary transmission. Aerosolization of MRSA can occur from the respiratory tract. In patients without chronic wounds or devices and intact skin, the nasopharynx becomes the primary site of persistent colonization and remains an ongoing source for endogenous infection with MRSA, but may be less important as a reservoir for secondary spread (von Eiff *et al.*, 2001). Nasopharyngeal colonization with MRSA can persist for years in the absence of specific therapy (Sanford *et al.*, 1994). It remains unproven as to whether MRSA strains are more virulent than susceptible strains, though increased resistance itself acts as a virulence factor and contributes to worse clinical outcomes by delayed initiation and decreased effectiveness of antimicrobial therapy.

Unlike enterococcal bacteremia, in which adverse consequences of delayed therapy may be difficult to demonstrate, untreated *S. aureus* bacteremia can be catastrophic. The responsibility falls to clinical laboratories to rapidly and accurately differentiate MRSA from susceptible *S. aureus* to optimize initial therapy and simultaneously decrease unnecessary vancomycin usage. Homogeneously expressing MRSA, which comprise the majority of endemic nosocomial isolates, are fairly well detected by standard disc diffusion and broth microdilution methods. Hetero-resistant strains, which may express methicillin resistance in as few as 1 in 10^8 colonies, pose a greater challenge. Expression of resistance is enhanced by neutral pH, lower temperature and high salt concentrations (Chambers, 1993). 2% NaCl supplementation facilitates detection of MRSA by disc diffusion on Mueller Hinton agar using standard National Committee for Clinical Laboratory Standards guidelines. Screen agar with 6 µg/mL of oxacillin and 4% NaCl has a sensitivity of close to 100% for detection of *mecA* strains (Chambers, 1993). Genotypic methods including PCR and nucleic acid hybridization are also ideally suited for detecting the highly conserved *mecA* gene in clinical isolates (Fluit *et al.*, 2001). PCR for *mecA* can also be applied directly to clinical specimens such as blood culture bottles.

Community Acquired MRSA

Early during the global MRSA epidemic it was recognized that MRSA colonization and infection could be identified in patients from the community at the time of their initial hospitalization. Usually some risk factor could be defined in these patients to account for their acquisition of MRSA. These risk factors include prior hospitalization or contact with a recently hospitalized or known MRSA infected patient, exposure to healthcare facilities as an outpatient or healthcare worker, significant prior antimicrobial exposures, and intravenous drug use (Layton *et al.*, 1995; Chambers, 2001). Long-term care facilities have become major reservoirs of MRSA colonized patients. Intravenous drug use was a major risk factor in many of the initial 1980's MRSA outbreaks in large U.S. urban hospitals (Saravolatz *et al.*, 1982). The mechanism of MRSA colonization among drug users may relate to sharing needles or other paraphernalia such as nasal straws, facilitating transmission of hospital acquired strains through the drug-using population. Such community-acquired strains are usually indistinguishable genetically and by resistance profiles from typical hospital multidrug-resistant MRSA and should be considered hospital associated even if they are not directly hospital acquired.

Beginning in 1999, several recent reports described true community MRSA infections in individuals, usually children, without any of the previously identified risk factors (Herold *et al.*, 1998; CDC, 1999; Chambers, 2001). These reports include descriptions of increased MRSA colonization rates in children in daycare centers in Texas as well as increased MRSA infections in otherwise healthy children hospitalized in Chicago (Adcock *et al.*, 1998; Herold *et al.*, 1998). More ominous are reports of 4 deaths among children in rural communities who presented with unsuspected MRSA infections, where delay of appropriate therapy contributed to the poor outcome (CDC, 1999). Unlike typical nosocomial MRSA, these isolates were often methicillin but not multidrug-resistant, and had genotypic profiles different than the predominant circulating MRSA clones. There have now been multiple additional descriptions of community MRSA, especially from pediatric populations. The initial origins of these community MRSA strains is unknown, but their emergence raises concern that the horizontal transfer of *mec* elements between strains, previously presumed to be an extremely rare event, may now be occurring more frequently. The recent sequencing of the *mecA* region from several community MRSA strains has demonstrated that the *mecA* cassettes in these strains are only 20 to 24 kb, and lack the other *mecA*-associated antimicrobial resistance genes found in typical hospital MRSA strains. These shorter *mecA* cassettes may facilitate easier horizontal transfer of beta-lactam resistance between staphylococci via bacteriophages or by other mechanisms (Ma *et al.*, 2002).

Strategies for Control of Nosocomial MRSA

Rates of MRSA vary widely from country to country, region to region and even from hospital to hospital (Panlilio *et al.*, 1992; Voss *et al.*, 1994). Thus, the strategies to limit nosocomial acquisition of MRSA must be individually designed to meet the needs of a particular institution. In institutions with very low rates of MRSA, strategies employing intensive surveillance and strict isolation procedures are clearly warranted to prevent the establishment of an endemic focus of MRSA. Where MRSA rates are very high, there is more controversy about how aggressively institutions should continue to pursue these costly measures to limit further spread (Herwaldt, 1999). Several consensus panels have published recommendations for control of MRSA, although not all of these recommendations are either appropriate or feasible for every health care facility (Report of a combined working party of the Hospital Infection Society and British Society for Antimicrobial Chemotherapy, 1990; Boyce *et al.*, 1994a; Goldmann *et al.*, 1996; Wenzel *et al.*, 1998).

Some components of MRSA control are applicable to all institutions (Table 3). These include optimization of laboratory procedures for identification of MRSA, review of microbiology data to identify all MRSA colonized or infected patients, mechanisms to continue to identify MRSA patients on transfer or discharge and readmission, use of hand washing or decontamination, and restriction of inappropriate antimicrobial usage. Numerous studies have now convincingly demonstrated an association between antibiotic use and MRSA, particularly use of 3rd generation cephalosporins and fluoroquinolones (Monnet, 1998; Diekema *et al.*, 2001; Monnet and Frimodt-Moller, 2001). Hospital formulary changes can also lead to decrease in MRSA rates (Landman *et al.*, 1999). Education of health care providers is also a critical component of any infection control program.

Other recommendations applicable to most institutions include some form of barrier precautions for MRSA (Herwaldt, 1999; Boyce, 2001). The U.S. Centers for Disease Control and Prevention recommends contact precautions for MRSA (Garner, 1996). This includes private rooms or cohorting of MRSA patients, gloves for contact with patient and their immediate environment as well as gowns if soilage of clothes is likely, and hand washing with antimicrobial soap. Not all MRSA patients are equally important reservoirs for dissemination of MRSA, and stratification of precautions based on risk of transmission may appropriate, especially where resources are limited. Barrier precautions alone have often been inadequate to control MRSA outbreaks (Herwaldt, 1999). Where endemic MRSA rates are extremely high, creation of an isolation ward may be necessary to protect newly admitted non-colonized patients.

Other procedures that may be useful include use of surveillance cultures. These can be helpful to assess prevalence rates, to identify MRSA colonized patients who are moving from high prevalence to low prevalence areas, and to reevaluate the status of known previously colonized, as on hospital readmission. Molecular epidemiology of nosocomial isolates may help to define the pattern of spread within or between institutions to help target control strategies. Screening of healthcare workers for chronic carriage may also be necessary to identify the source of prolonged, unexplained outbreaks.

The role of MRSA decolonization continues to evolve. Decolonization strategies have included short courses of oral antimicrobial combinations, generally novobiocin, ciprofloxacin or trimethoprim-sulfamethoxazole plus rifampin (Mulligan *et al.*, 1993). Bacitracin, and more recently mupirocin are used topically for selective nasopharyngeal decolonization. Oral regimens may be effective for clearing nasopharyngeal colonization but are less effective at other sites and may lead to increased resistance to the agents used. Mupirocin can be effective in short-term clearance of nasopharyngeal colonization as well as prevention of MRSA wound infection in patients at high risk, such as those undergoing cardiothoracic surgery (Kluytmans *et al.*, 1996b). Intermittent mupirocin has also decreased rates of MRSA infection in MRSA-colonized hemodialysis patients (Kluytmans *et al.*, 1996a). Clearance of nasopharyngeal colonization by mupirocin also results in clearing of hand carriage of MRSA (Reagan *et al.*, 1991). Unfortunately, resistance to mupirocin can develop following prolonged use, and nosocomial transmission of plasmid-mediated mupirocin resistance can occur (Morton *et al.*, 1995). Decolonization of patients and healthcare workers may be most useful during epidemics but is not necessarily indicated for all MRSA patients.

Glycopeptide Resistant *S. aureus* Strains

Ever since the emergence of VRE in 1989, physicians have pondered the catastrophic implications of glycopeptide resistance emerging in MRSA (Edmond *et al.*, 1996). Vancomycin resistance in coagulase-negative staphylococci was first reported in 1987, and there are now numerous descriptions of such isolates (Schwalbe *et al.*, 1987). Emergence of glycopeptide resistance in coagulase-negative staphylococci is species related, occurring most often in *S. haemolyticus* and occasionally in *S. epidermidis* (Froggatt *et al.*, 1989; Fraimow and Courvalin, 2000). Vancomycin- resistant *S. haemolyticus* and *S. epidermidis* are readily selected *in vitro* by serial passage on vancomycin or teicoplanin, and strains with vancomycin MICs as high as 128 µg/mL have been described. Despite relative ease of selection *in vitro*, glycopeptide resistance is still extremely uncommon among clinical isolates although the proportion of strains with MIC's of 4 µg/mL is increasing (Sahm *et al.*, 1999; Diekema *et al.*, 2001). Investigators have also been able to serially passage *S. aureus* strains to select mutants with reduced vancomycin susceptibility, but until recently these observations were not considered very significant as no similar clinical isolates had been reported (Daum *et al.*, 1992; Sieradzki and Tomasz, 1997). The enterococcal vancomycin resistance gene cluster *vanA* has been successfully transferred to *S. aureus in vitro* (Noble *et al.*, 1992).

The first clinical isolate of *S. aureus* with reduced glycopeptide susceptibility was reported from Japan in 1997 (Hiramatsu *et al.*, 1997b). Since that time there have been multiple similar strains reported from the U.S. as well as from Europe and the Far East, some described in association with clinical failure of vancomycin therapy but others found only in retrospective surveys of collected isolates (CDC, 1997b; CDC, 1997c; Tenover *et al.*, 2001). These strains, which have reduced susceptibility to both vancomycin and teicoplanin, are called either vancomycin intermediate *S. aureus* (VISA) or glycopeptide intermediate *S. aureus* (GISA). MIC's to vancomycin are typically 8-16 µg/mL. Strains with vancomycin MICs 32 µg/mL are termed VRSA. Great confusion still remains over the exact definition of this form of glycopeptide resistance, the optimal testing methodology to identify these strains, and their clinical importance, particularly for strains only identified retrospectively (Tenover *et al.*, 2001).

Despite these controversies, several observations can be made about clinical GISA strains. The initial Japanese isolate Mu50 and several of the U.S. isolates appear to have evolved from genetically identical glycopeptide-susceptible MRSA in patients with long-term vancomycin exposures, and were associated with vancomycin failure (CDC, 1997b; CDC, 1997c; Hiramatsu *et al.*, 1997b). In animal models such strains with MIC's of 8 μg/mL are also associated with vancomycin failure. There is as yet no evidence of secondary transmission of GISA strains to other patients. More prevalent than these GISA strains are so-called hetero-resistant GISA isolates. Hetero-resistant strains, which have been reported in as many as 1.3% of MRSA in one survey from Japan, are strains from which subpopulations can be reproducibly selected that will grow on Brain Heart agar containing progressively higher vancomycin concentrations (Hiramatsu *et al.*, 1997a). Stable GISA strains can be readily selected *in vitro* from more resistant subpopulations of hetero-resistant strains, but whether hetero-resistance represents an early stage of evolution into a GISA strain is unknown. Although clinical GISA strains have been MRSA, GISA can be also generated *in vitro* from methicillin-susceptible *S. aureus*. It is also unclear how "new" GISA are. Screening of historical *S. aureus* strain collections has identified phenotypically similar strains from as far back as the early 1980's (Bierbaum *et al.*, 1999). The phenomenon of "vancomycin failure" in treatment of *S. aureus* infections is well described, and perhaps subpopulations of MRSA with reduced susceptibility to might explain the relatively high rate of these clinical failures. Guidelines for the management of patients with confirmed or suspected GISA have recently been published (CDC, 1997a).

The specific mechanisms resulting in reduced glycopeptide susceptibility in GISA have not been elaborated, but several observations about these strains have been reported. GISA strains do not contain genes analogous to those conferring acquired enterococcal vancomycin resistance. Phenotypically, most strains demonstrate slow growth rates, heterogeneous colony morphology on vancomycin-containing media, thickened cell walls, altered lysostaphin sensitivity, and often a paradoxical hyper-susceptibility to beta-lactams (Tenover *et al.*, 2001). In the Japanese strain Mu50 and some of the Japanese hetero-resistant isolates there is also evidence of altered PBP expression, particularly increased levels of PBP2 and PBP2', and altered cell wall precursors (Hanaki *et al.*, 1998a; 1998b). Others have reported evidence for decreased cross-linking in the cell wall. All these observations are consistent with a mechanism in which GISA strains produce thickened cell wall with excess distal vancomycin binding sites that can then trap vancomycin prior to it's reaching it's target in nascent peptidoglycan adjacent to the bacterial membrane (Fraimow and Courvalin, 2000). Enhanced expression of PBPs may also decrease the amount of available target for vancomycin by more efficient transpeptidation during peptidoglycan synthesis.

Recently, the first clinical high level vancomycin resistant MRSA strain has been described (CDC, 2002). This strain, isolated from a dialysis patient receiving vancomycin therapy for an MRSA catheter infection, was reported to have an MIC to vancomycin of > 32 µg/mL and has also been found to contain the *vanA* enterococcal vancomycin resistance gene. Thus far, however, transfer of *vanA* to *S. aureus in vivo* appears to be an extremely rare event.

Treatment of MRSA and Other Multidrug-Resistant Staphylococci

Vancomycin currently remains the primary choice for treatment of serious infections due to MRSA, although this may change with further emergence of GISA strains and development of better anti-staphylococcal agents. Vancomycin is bactericidal against most *S. aureus*, but killing is less rapid and the time to defervescence more prolonged compared to β-lactams in therapy of non-MRSA infection (Chambers, 1997). It is not unusual for bacteremia to persist for over a week in patients on vancomycin for MRSA endovascular infections, and treatment failure rates may approach 20% (Levine *et al.*, 1991). Despite apparent *in vitro* susceptibility to some β-lactams, *S. aureus* strains resistant to oxacillin must be presumed to be resistant to all currently available β-lactam agents. Newer β-lactams are in development that are specifically targeted to bind to PBP2' and are active against MRSA *in vivo* (Chamberland *et al.*, 2001).

Most MRSA strains are also resistant to multiple other drug classes (Table 4). Tetracycline, erythromycin and tobramycin resistance determinants are often incorporated into the *mec* gene cluster (Chambers, 2001). Tetracycline resistance in staphylococci is primarily mediated by the pT181-associated TetK efflux pump or less commonly by TetL and TetM. Minocycline remains active against most tetracycline resistant strains except the rare strains containing TetM. Minocycline can be bactericidal for MRSA, and can be used as an alternative for treatment of less severe MRSA infections (Yuk *et al.*, 1991). ErmA, B and C, especially the *mec* associated ErmA methylases, are widely distributed among *S. aureus*, as is the erythromycin efflux pump MsrA (Schmitz *et al.*, 2000). Some MRSA strains with inducible *erm* genes are clindamycin susceptible *in vitro*, but evolution to constitutive *erm* expression leads to cross-resistance to clindamycin. Aminoglycoside inactivating enzymes, particularly AAC(6')—APH(2"), are varyingly distributed in MRSA, but many nosocomial strains still remain gentamicin susceptible (Table 4). In susceptible strains gentamicin is rapidly bactericidal but cannot be used alone, due to rapid emergence of small colony variant gentamicin-resistant mutants (Miller *et al.*, 1978).

When first introduced, ciprofloxacin was active against most MRSA strains, but resistance rapidly developed with increasing usage (Daum *et al.*, 1990). Newer quinolones with enhanced gram-positive activity including levofloxacin, gatifloxacin and moxifloxacin are very active against ciprofloxacin susceptible strains, but resistance to these agents rapidly develops in strains already partially or fully ciprofloxacin resistant. Quinolone resistance occurs through sequential selection of multiple mutations primarily in topoisomerase IV (usually *grlA*) but also in DNA gyrase (*gyrA*) (Ng *et al.*, 1996; Chambers, 1997). Low-level resistance to some quinolones can also occur by up-regulation of an intrinsic staphylococcal NorA efflux pump (Kaatz *et al.*, 1993). When quinolones are used for treatment of quinolone-susceptible MRSA, rifampin is often added to prevent emergence of resistance. Rifampin is a potent, bactericidal anti-staphylococcal agent active against most MRSA, but high-level resistant mutants with alterations in ribosomal polymerase are selected at high frequency. Rifampin is primarily combined with other agents including vancomycin, quinolones or trimethoprim-sulfamethoxazole to either enhance killing or prevent emergence of resistance (Chambers, 1997). In many hospitals, over 70% of MRSA strains are still susceptible to trimethoprim-sulfamethoxazole (Diekema *et al.*, 2001). This agent is inferior to vancomycin in animal models of endovascular infection but remains an alternative to vancomycin for treatment of less serious infections and can also be given orally (de Gorgolas *et al.*, 1995). Fusidic acid, a protein synthesis inhibitor available in Europe but not the U.S., can be used in anti-staphylococcal combination therapy but resistance develops when it is used alone.

With the emergence of GISA strains, additional potent anti-staphylococcal agents are desperately needed. The new gram-positive agents quinupristin-dalfopristin and linezolid, described in detail above, are active against *S. aureus* including MRSA. Quinupristin-dalfopristin is bactericidal against *S. aureus* strains possessing resistance to neither of the streptogramin components. However, most MRSA already possess inducible *erm* methylases mediating cross resistance to streptogramin B, thus constitutive expression of *erm* will result in streptogramin B resistance and often loss of bactericidal activity. Streptogramin A inactivating genes (*vatA*, *vatB*, and *vatC*) and streptogramin efflux pumps (*vgaA* and *vgaB*) are less common than *erm* methylases, but are also increasingly described in staphylococci (Lina *et al.*, 1999). Streptogramin A and B resistance genes can both be carried on the same plasmid (Allignet *et al.*, 1998). Strains carrying resistance to both streptogramin components will be resistant to quinupristin-dalfopristin. Linezolid has been highly active against nearly all MRSA strains *in vitro* and in clinical trails, but is also generally bacteriostatic (Diekema and Jones, 2001). Linezolid resistance has also evolved *in vivo* by mutations in the same region V of the 23S ribosome described in linezolid-resistant enterococci (Tsiodras *et al.*, 2001). Both linezolid and quinupristin-dalfopristin are increasingly being used for treatment of serious *S. aureus* infections including bacteremia, endocarditis, pneumonia and osteomyelitis in patients failing or intolerant of vancomycin, and comparative trials are ongoing to evaluate their role as primary therapy for MRSA. The lipopeptide daptomycin has also been used for MRSA infections in clinical trials (Tally and DeBruin, 2000).

Conclusion

The multi-resistant gram-positive pathogens VRE and MRSA have continued to increase in prevalence in the hospital and chronic care setting, and MRSA infections are now also increasingly reported in the community. Emergence of resistance in these pathogens is closely associated with antimicrobial usage, and antibiotic restriction is a critical component of programs to limit their spread. Treatment of MRSA and VRE is limited by their sequential accumulation of multiple resistance traits, some of which are clustered on transferable resistance elements and others of which are readily selected *in vivo*. The newly released gram-positive antibiotics linezolid and quinupristin-dalfopristin are active against these organisms, but use of these agents needs be monitored carefully to preserve their effectiveness.

References

Aarestrup, F.M. 1995. Occurrence of glycopeptide resistance among *Enterococcus faecium* isolates from conventional and ecological poultry farms. Microb. Drug Resist. 1: 255-257.

Aarestrup, F.M., Seyfarth, A.M., Emborg, H.D., Pedersen, K., Hendriksen, R.S., and Bager, F. 2001. Effect of abolishment of the use of antimicrobial agents for growth promotion on occurrence of antimicrobial resistance in fecal enterococci from food animals in Denmark. Antimicrob. Agents Chemother. 45: 2054-2059.

Adcock, P.M., Pastor, P., Medley, F., Patterson, J.E., and Murphy, T.V. 1998. Methicillin-resistant *Staphylococcus aureus* in two child care centers. J. Infect. Dis. 178: 577-580.

Allignet, J., Liassine, N., and el Solh, N. 1998. Characterization of a staphylococcal plasmid related to pUB110 and carrying two novel genes, *vatC* and *vgbB*, encoding resistance to streptogramins A and B and similar antibiotics. Antimicrob. Agents Chemother. 42: 1794-1798.

Archer, G.L., and Niemeyer, D.M. 1994. Origin and evolution of DNA associated with resistance to methicillin in staphylococci. Trends Microbiol. 2: 343-347.

Arias, C.A., Courvalin, P., and Reynolds, P.E. 2000. *vanC* cluster of vancomycin-resistant *Enterococcus gallinarum* BM4174. Antimicrob. Agents Chemother. 44: 1660-1666.

Arthur, M., Molinas, C., and Courvalin, P. 1992. The VanS-VanR two-component regulatory system controls synthesis of depsipeptide peptidoglycan precursors in *Enterococcus faecium* BM4147. J. Bacteriol. 174: 2582-2591.

Arthur, M., Molinas, C., Depardieu, F., and Courvalin, P. 1993. Characterization of Tn*1546*, a Tn*3*-related transposon conferring glycopeptide resistance by synthesis of depsipeptide peptidoglycan precursors in *Enterococcus faecium* BM4147. J. Bacteriol. 175: 117-127.

Arthur, M., and Quintiliani, R., Jr. 2001. Regulation of VanA- and VanB-type glycopeptide resistance in enterococci. Antimicrob. Agents Chemother. 45: 375-381.

Arthur, M., Reynolds, P., and Courvalin, P. 1996. Glycopeptide resistance in enterococci. Trends Microbiol. 4: 401-407.

Barrett, F.F., McGehee, R.F., Jr., and Finland, M. 1968. Methicillin-resistant *Staphylococcus aureus* at Boston City Hospital. Bacteriologic and epidemiologic observations. N. Engl. J. Med. 279: 441-448.

Berger-Bachi, B., Strassle, A., and Kayser, F.H. 1986. Characterization of an isogenic set of methicillin-resistant and susceptible mutants of *Staphylococcus aureus*. Eur. J. Clin. Microbiol. 5: 697-701.

Bierbaum, G., Fuchs, K., Lenz, W., Szekat, C., and Sahl, H.G. 1999. Presence of *Staphylococcus aureus* with reduced susceptibility to vancomycin in Germany. Eur. J. Clin. Microbiol. Infect Dis. 18: 691-696.

Bonten, M.J., Slaughter, S., Ambergen, A.W., Hayden, M.K., van Voorhis, J., Nathan, C., and Weinstein, R.A. 1998. The role of "colonization pressure" in the spread of vancomycin- resistant enterococci: an important infection control variable. Arch. Intern. Med. 158: 1127-1132.

Boyce, J.M. 2001. MRSA patients: proven methods to treat colonization and infection. J. Hosp. Infect. 48 Suppl A: S9-S14.

Boyce, J.M., Jackson, M.M., Pugliese, G., Batt, M.D., Fleming, D., Garner, J.S., Hartstein, A.I., Kauffman, C.A., Simmons, M., and Weinstein, R. 1994a. Methicillin-resistant *Staphylococcus aureus* (MRSA): a briefing for acute care hospitals and nursing facilities. The AHA Technical Panel on Infections Within Hospitals. Infect. Control Hosp. Epidemiol. 15: 105-115.

Boyce, J.M., Opal, S.M., Chow, J.W., Zervos, M.J., Potter-Bynoe, G., Sherman, C.B., Romulo, R.L., Fortna, S., and Medeiros, A.A. 1994b. Outbreak of multidrug-resistant *Enterococcus faecium* with transferable *vanB* class vancomycin resistance. J. Clin. Microbiol. 32: 1148-1153.

Boyce, J.M., Opal, S.M., Potter-Bynoe, G., LaForge, R.G., Zervos, M.J., Furtado, G., Victor, G., and Medeiros, A.A. 1992. Emergence and nosocomial transmission of ampicillin-resistant enterococci. Antimicrob. Agents Chemother. 36: 1032-1039.

Boyce, J.M., Potter-Bynoe, G., Chenevert, C., and King, T. 1997. Environmental contamination due to methicillin-resistant *Staphylococcus aureus*: possible infection control implications. Infect. Control Hosp. Epidemiol. 18: 622-627.

Brisse, S., Fluit, A.C., Wagner, U., Heisig, P., Milatovic, D., Verhoef, J., Scheuring, S., Kohrer, K., and Schmitz, F.J. 1999. Association of alterations in ParC and GyrA proteins with resistance of clinical isolates of *Enterococcus faecium* to nine different fluoroquinolones. Antimicrob. Agents Chemother. 43: 2513-2516.

Bugg, T.D., Dutka-Malen, S., Arthur, M., Courvalin, P., and Walsh, C.T. 1991. Identification of vancomycin resistance protein VanA as a D-alanine:D- alanine ligase of altered substrate specificity. Biochemistry. 30: 2017-2021.

Calderwood, S.A., Wennersten, C., Moellering, R.C., Jr., Kunz, L.J., and Krogstad, D.J. 1977. Resistance to six aminoglycosidic aminocyclitol antibiotics among enterococci: prevalence, evolution, and relationship to synergism with penicillin. Antimicrob. Agents Chemother. 12: 401-405.

Carias, L.L., Rudin, S.D., Donskey, C.J., and Rice, L.B. 1998. Genetic linkage and cotransfer of a novel, *vanB*-containing transposon (Tn*5382*) and a low-affinity penicillin-binding protein 5 gene in a clinical vancomycin-resistant *Enterococcus faecium* isolate. J. Bacteriol. 180: 4426-4434.

Casadewall, B., and Courvalin, P. 1999. Characterization of the *vanD* glycopeptide resistance gene cluster from *Enterococcus faecium* BM4339. J. Bacteriol. 181: 3644-3648.

CDC. 1997a. Interim guidelines for prevention and control of staphylococcal infection associated with reduced susceptibility to vancomycin. MMWR Morb. Mortal. Wkly. Rep. 46: 626-628, 635.

CDC. 1997b. *Staphylococcus aureus* with reduced susceptibility to vancomycin—United States, 1997. MMWR Morb. Mortal. Wkly. Rep. 46: 765-766.

CDC. 1997c. Update: *Staphylococcus aureus* with reduced susceptibility to vancomycin- -United States, 1997. MMWR Morb. Mortal. Wkly. Rep. 46: 813-815.

CDC. 1999. From the Centers for Disease Control and Prevention. Four pediatric deaths from community-acquired methicillin-resistant *Staphylococcus aureus*—Minnesota and North Dakota, 1997-1999. J.A.M.A. 282: 1123-1125.

CDC. 2002. *Staphylococcus aureus* resistant to vancomycin—United States, 2002. MMWR Morb. Mortal. Wkly. Rep. 51: 565-567.

Chamberland, S., Blais, J., Hoang, M., Dinh, C., Cotter, D., Bond, E., Gannon, C., Park, C., Malouin, F., and Dudley, M.N. 2001. *In vitro* activities of RWJ-54428 (MC-02,479) against multiresistant gram-positive bacteria. Antimicrob. Agents Chemother. 45: 1422-1430.

Chambers, H.F. 1993. Detection of methicillin-resistant staphylococci. Infect. Dis. Clin. North Am. 7: 425-433.

Chambers, H.F. 1997. Methicillin resistance in staphylococci: molecular and biochemical basis and clinical implications. Clin. Microbiol. Rev. 10: 781-791.

Chambers, H.F. 2001. The changing epidemiology of *Staphylococcus aureus*? Emerg. Infect. Dis. 7: 178-182.

Chambers, H.F., Sachdeva, M., and Kennedy, S. 1990. Binding affinity for penicillin-binding protein 2a correlates with *in vivo* activity of beta-lactam antibiotics against methicillin-resistant *Staphylococcus aureus*. J. Infect. Dis. 162: 705-710.

Chow, J.W. 2000. Aminoglycoside resistance in enterococci. Clin. Infect. Dis. 31: 586-589.

Coque, T.M., Arduino, R.C., and Murray, B.E. 1995. High-level resistance to aminoglycosides: comparison of community and nosocomial fecal isolates of enterococci. Clin. Infect. Dis. 20: 1048-1051.

Courvalin, P., Carlier, C., and Collatz, E. 1980. Plasmid-mediated resistance to aminocyclitol antibiotics in group D streptococci. J. Bacteriol. 143: 541-551.

Daum, R.S., Gupta, S., Sabbagh, R., and Milewski, W.M. 1992. Characterization of *Staphylococcus aureus* isolates with decreased susceptibility to vancomycin and teicoplanin: isolation and purification of a constitutively produced protein associated with decreased susceptibility. J. Infect. Dis. 166: 1066-1072.

Daum, T.E., Schaberg, D.R., Terpenning, M.S., Sottile, W.S., and Kauffman, C.A. 1990. Increasing resistance of *Staphylococcus aureus* to ciprofloxacin. Antimicrob. Agents Chemother. 34: 1862-1863.

de Gorgolas, M., Aviles, P., Verdejo, C., and Fernandez Guerrero, M.L. 1995. Treatment of experimental endocarditis due to methicillin-susceptible or methicillin-resistant *Staphylococcus aureus* with trimethoprim- sulfamethoxazole and antibiotics that inhibit cell wall synthesis. Antimicrob. Agents Chemother. 39: 953-957.

de Lencastre, H., and Tomasz, A. 1994. Reassessment of the number of auxiliary genes essential for expression of high-level methicillin resistance in *Staphylococcus aureus*. Antimicrob. Agents Chemother. 38: 2590-2598.

Diekema, D.J., and Jones, R.N. 2001. Oxazolidinone antibiotics. Lancet. 358: 1975-1982.

Diekema, D.J., Pfaller, M.A., Schmitz, F.J., Smayevsky, J., Bell, J., Jones, R.N., and Beach, M. 2001. Survey of infections due to *Staphylococcus* species: frequency of occurrence and antimicrobial susceptibility of isolates collected in the United States, Canada, Latin America, Europe, and the Western Pacific region for the SENTRY Antimicrobial Surveillance Program, 1997- 1999. Clin. Infect. Dis. 32 Suppl 2: S114-S132.

Donskey, C.J., Chowdhry, T.K., Hecker, M.T., Hoyen, C.K., Hanrahan, J.A., Hujer, A.M., Hutton-Thomas, R.A., Whalen, C.C., Bonomo, R.A., and Rice, L.B. 2000. Effect of antibiotic therapy on the density of vancomycin-resistant enterococci in the stool of colonized patients. N. Engl. J. Med. 343: 1925-1932.

Donskey, C.J., Hume, M.E., Callaway, T.R., Das, S.M., Hoyen, C.K., and Rice, L.B. 2001. Inhibition of vancomycin-resistant enterococci by an *in vitro* continuous-flow competitive exclusion culture containing human stool flora. J. Infect. Dis. 184: 1624-1627.

Edmond, M.B., Wenzel, R.P., and Pasculle, A.W. 1996. Vancomycin-resistant *Staphylococcus aureus*: perspectives on measures needed for control. Ann. Intern. Med. 124: 329-334.

Edmond, M.B., Wallace, S.E., McLish, D.K., Pfaller, M.A., Jones, R.N., and Wenzel, R.P. 1999. Nosocomial bloodstream infections in United States hospitals: a three-year analysis. Clin. Infect. Dis 29: 239-244

Elsner, H.A., Sobottka, I., Mack, D., Claussen, M., Laufs, R., and Wirth, R. 2000. Virulence factors of *Enterococcus faecalis* and *Enterococcus faecium* blood culture isolates. Eur. J. Clin .Microbiol. Infect. Dis. 19: 39-42.

European Antimicrobial Resistance Surveillance System. EARSS Database. 2002. Available from URL: http://www.earss.rivm.nl/PAGINA/interwebsite/home_earss.html.

Evers, S., Casadewall, B., Charles, M., Dutka-Malen, S., Galimand, M., and Courvalin, P. 1996. Evolution of structure and substrate specificity in D-alanine:D-alanine ligases and related enzymes. J. Mol. Evol. 42: 706-712.

Evers, S., and Courvalin, P. 1996. Regulation of VanB-type vancomycin resistance gene expression by the VanS(B)-VanR(B) two-component regulatory system in *Enterococcus faecalis* V583. J. Bacteriol. 178: 1302-1309.

Ferretti, J.J., Gilmore, K.S., and Courvalin, P. 1986. Nucleotide sequence analysis of the gene specifying the bifunctional 6'-aminoglycoside acetyltransferase 2"-aminoglycoside phosphotransferase enzyme in *Streptococcus faecalis* and identification and cloning of gene regions specifying the two activities. J. Bacteriol. 167: 631-638.

Fines, M., Perichon, B., Reynolds, P., Sahm, D.F., and Courvalin, P. 1999. VanE, a new type of acquired glycopeptide resistance in *Enterococcus faecalis* BM4405. Antimicrob. Agents Chemother. 43: 2161-2164.

Fluit, A.C., Visser, M.R., and Schmitz, F.J. 2001. Molecular detection of antimicrobial resistance. Clin. Microbiol. Rev. 14: 836-871.

Fraimow, H.S., and Courvalin, P. 2000. Resistance to Glycopeptides in Gram Positive Pathogens. In: Gram-Positive Pathogens. V. A.

Fischetti, R. P. Novick, J. J. Ferretti, D. A. Portnoy, and J. I. Rood, eds. ASM Press, Washington, D.C. p. 621-634.

Fraimow, H.S., and Venuti, E. 1992. Inconsistent bactericidal activity of triple-combination therapy with vancomycin, ampicillin, and gentamicin against vancomycin-resistant, highly ampicillin-resistant *Enterococcus faecium*. Antimicrob. Agents Chemother. 36: 1563-1566.

Fridkin, S.K., and Gaynes, R.P. 1999. Antimicrobial resistance in intensive care units. Clin. Chest Med. 20:303-16.

Fridkin, S.K., Edwards, J.R., Courval, J.M., Hill, H., Tenover, F.C., Lawton, R., Gaynes, R.P., and McGowan, J.E., Jr. 2001. The effect of vancomycin and third-generation cephalosporins on prevalence of vancomycin-resistant enterococci in 126 U.S. adult intensive care units. Ann. Intern. Med. 135: 175-183.

Froggatt, J.W., Johnston, J.L., Galetto, D.W., and Archer, G.L. 1989. Antimicrobial resistance in nosocomial isolates of *Staphylococcus haemolyticus*. Antimicrob. Agents Chemother. 33: 460-466.

Garner, J.S. 1996. Guideline for isolation precautions in hospitals. The Hospital Infection Control Practices Advisory Committee. Infect. Control Hosp. Epidemiol. 17: 53-80.

Gold, H.S., Unal, S., Cercenado, E., Thauvin-Eliopoulos, C., Eliopoulos, G.M., Wennersten, C.B., and Moellering, R.C., Jr. 1993. A gene conferring resistance to vancomycin but not teicoplanin in isolates of *Enterococcus faecalis* and *Enterococcus faecium* demonstrates homology with *vanB, vanA*, and *vanC* genes of enterococci. Antimicrob. Agents Chemother. 37: 1604-1609.

Goldmann, D.A., Weinstein, R.A., Wenzel, R.P., Tablan, O.C., Duma, R.J., Gaynes, R.P., Schlosser, J., and Martone, W.J. 1996. Strategies to Prevent and Control the Emergence and Spread of Antimicrobial-Resistant Microorganisms in Hospitals. A challenge to hospital leadership. J. Am. Med. Asoc. 275: 234-240.

Gonzales, R.D., Schreckenberger, P.C., Graham, M.B., Kelkar, S., DenBesten, K., and Quinn, J.P. 2001. Infections due to vancomycin-resistant *Enterococcus faecium* resistant to linezolid. Lancet. 357: 1179.

Goossens, H. 1998. Spread of vancomycin-resistant enterococci: differences between the United States and Europe. Infect. Control Hosp. Epidemiol. 19: 546-551.

Grayson, M.L., Eliopoulos, G.M., Wennersten, C.B., Ruoff, K.L., De Girolami, P.C., Ferraro, M.J., and Moellering, R.C., Jr. 1991. Increasing resistance to beta-lactam antibiotics among clinical isolates of *Enterococcus faecium*: a 22-year review at one institution. Antimicrob. Agents Chemother. 35: 2180-2184.

Hanaki, H., Kuwahara-Arai, K., Boyle-Vavra, S., Daum, R.S., Labischinski, H., and Hiramatsu, K. 1998a. Activated cell-wall synthesis is associated with vancomycin resistance in methicillin-resistant *Staphylococcus aureus* clinical strains Mu3 and Mu50. J. Antimicrob. Chemother. 42: 199-209.

Hanaki, H., Labischinski, H., Inaba, Y., Kondo, N., Murakami, H., and Hiramatsu, K. 1998b. Increase in glutamine-non-amidated muropeptides in the peptidoglycan of vancomycin-resistant *Staphylococcus aureus* strain Mu50. J. Antimicrob. Chemother. 42: 315-320.

Handwerger, S., Perlman, D.C., Altarac, D., and McAuliffe, V. 1992. Concomitant high-level vancomycin and penicillin resistance in clinical isolates of enterococci. Clin. Infect. Dis. 14: 655-661.

Handwerger, S., and Tomasz, A. 1985. Antibiotic tolerance among clinical isolates of bacteria. Rev. Infect. Dis. 7: 368-386.

Hartman, B.J., and Tomasz, A. 1984. Low-affinity penicillin-binding protein associated with beta-lactam resistance in *Staphylococcus aureus*. J. Bacteriol. 158: 513-516.

Herold, B.C., Immergluck, L.C., Maranan, M.C., Lauderdale, D.S., Gaskin, R.E., Boyle-Vavra, S., Leitch, C.D., and Daum, R.S. 1998. Community-acquired methicillin-resistant *Staphylococcus aureus* in children with no identified predisposing risk. J. Am. Med. Assoc. 279: 593-598.

Herwaldt, L.A. 1999. Control of methicillin-resistant *Staphylococcus aureus* in the hospital setting. Am. J. Med. 106: 11S-18S.

Hospital Infection Control Practices Advisory Committee. 1995. Recommendations for preventing the spread of vancomycin resistance. Infect. Control Hosp. Epidemiol. 16: 105-113.

Hiramatsu, K., Aritaka, N., Hanaki, H., Kawasaki, S., Hosoda, Y., Hori, S., Fukuchi, Y., and Kobayashi, I. 1997a. Dissemination in Japanese hospitals of strains of *Staphylococcus aureus* heterogeneously resistant to vancomycin. Lancet. 350: 1670-1673.

Hiramatsu, K., Hanaki, H., Ino, T., Yabuta, K., Oguri, T., and Tenover, F.C. 1997b. Methicillin-resistant *Staphylococcus aureus* clinical strain with reduced vancomycin susceptibility. J. Antimicrob. Chemother. 40: 135-136.

Hospital Infections Program, National Center for Infectious Diseases. 1999. National Nosocomial Infections Surveillance (NNIS) System report, data summary from January 1990-May 1999, issued June 1999. Am. J. Infect. Control. 27: 520-532.

Jensen, L.B., Hammerum, A.M., and Aarestrup, F.M. 2000. Linkage of *vat(E)* and *erm(B)* in streptogamin-resistant *Enterococcus faecium* isolates from Europe. Antimicrob. Agents Chemother. 44: 2231-2232.

Jevons, M., Coe, A., and Parker, M. 1963. Methicillin resistance in staphylcocci. Lancet. i: 904-907.

Kaatz, G.W., Seo, S.M., and Ruble, C.A. 1993. Efflux-mediated fluoroquinolone resistance in *Staphylococcus aureus*. Antimicrob. Agents Chemother. 37: 1086-1094.

Kao, S.J., You, I., Clewell, D.B., Donabedian, S.M., Zervos, M.J., Petrin, J., Shaw, K.J., and Chow, J.W. 2000. Detection of the high-level aminoglycoside resistance gene *aph(2")-Ib* in *Enterococcus faecium*. Antimicrob. Agents Chemother. 44: 2876-2879.

Kirst, H.A., Thompson, D.G., and Nicas, T.I. 1998. Historical yearly usage of vancomycin. Antimicrob. Agents Chemother.42: 1303-1304.

Klare, I., Heier, H., Claus, H., and Witte, W. 1993. Environmental strains of *Enterococcus faecium* with inducible high-level resistance to glycopeptides. FEMS Microbiol. Lett. 80: 23-29.

Kluytmans, J.A., Manders, M.J., van Bommel, E., and Verbrugh, H. 1996a. Elimination of nasal carriage of *Staphylococcus aureus* in hemodialysis patients. Infect. Control Hosp. Epidemiol. 17: 793-797.

Kluytmans, J.A., Mouton, J.W., VandenBergh, M.F., Manders, M.J., Maat, A.P., Wagenvoort, J.H., Michel, M.F., and Verbrugh, H.A. 1996b. Reduction of surgical-site infections in cardiothoracic surgery by elimination of nasal carriage of *Staphylococcus aureus*. Infect. Control Hosp. Epidemiol. 17: 780-785.

Kreiswirth, B., Kornblum, J., Arbeit, R.D., Eisner, W., Maslow, J.N., McGeer, A., Low, D.E., and Novick, R.P. 1993. Evidence for a clonal origin of methicillin resistance in *Staphylococcus aureus*. Science. 259: 227-230.

Lai, K.K., Fontecchio, S.A., Kelley, A.L., Melvin, Z.S., and Baker, S. 1997. The epidemiology of fecal carriage of vancomycin-resistant enterococci. Infect. Control Hosp. Epidemiol. 18: 762-765.

Lai, K.K., Kelley, A.L., Melvin, Z.S., Belliveau, P.P., and Fontecchio, S.A. 1998. Failure to eradicate vancomycin-resistant enterococci in a university hospital and the cost of barrier precautions. Infect. Control Hosp. Epidemiol. 19: 647-652.

Landman, D., Chockalingam, M., and Quale, J.M. 1999. Reduction in the incidence of methicillin-resistant *Staphylococcus aureus* and ceftazidime-resistant *Klebsiella pneumoniae* following changes in a hospital antibiotic formulary. Clin. Infect. Dis. 28: 1062-1066.

Lautenbach, E., Schuster, M.G., Bilker, W.B., and Brennan, P.J. 1998. The role of chloramphenicol in the treatment of bloodstream infection due to vancomycin-resistant *Enterococcus*. Clin. Infect. Dis. 27: 1259-1265.

Layton, M.C., Hierholzer, W.J., Jr., and Patterson, J.E. 1995. The evolving epidemiology of methicillin-resistant *Staphylococcus aureus* at a university hospital. Infect. Control Hosp. Epidemiol. 16: 12-17.

Levine, D.P., Fromm, B.S., and Reddy, B.R. 1991. Slow response to vancomycin or vancomycin plus rifampin in methicillin- resistant *Staphylococcus aureus* endocarditis. Ann. Intern. Med. 115: 674-680.

Ligozzi, M., Lo Cascio, G., and Fontana, R. 1998. *vanA* gene cluster in a vancomycin-resistant clinical isolate of *Bacillus circulans*. Antimicrob. Agents Chemother. 42: 2055-2059.

Lina, G., Quaglia, A., Reverdy, M.E., Leclercq, R., Vandenesch, F., and Etienne, J. 1999. Distribution of genes encoding resistance to macrolides, lincosamides, and streptogramins among staphylococci. Antimicrob. Agents Chemother. 43: 1062-1066.

Linden, P.K., Moellering, R.C., Jr., Wood, C.A., Rehm, S.J., Flaherty, J., Bompart, F., and Talbot, G.H. 2001. Treatment of vancomycin-resistant *Enterococcus faecium* infections with quinupristin/dalfopristin. Clin. Infect. Dis. 33: 1816-1823.

Low, D.E., Keller, N., Barth, A., and Jones, R.N. 2001. Clinical prevalence, antimicrobial susceptibility, and geographic resistance patterns of enterococci: results from the SENTRY Antimicrobial Surveillance Program, 1997-1999. Clin. Infect. Dis. 32 Suppl. 2: S133-S145.

Lyon, B.R., and Skurray, R. 1987. Antimicrobial resistance of *Staphylococcus aureus*: genetic basis. Microbiol. Rev. 51: 88-134.

Marshall, C.G., Broadhead, G., Leskiw, B.K., and Wright, G.D. 1997. D-Ala-D-Ala ligases from glycopeptide antibiotic-producing organisms are highly homologous to the enterococcal vancomycin-resistance ligases VanA and VanB. Proc. Natl. Acad. Sci. USA. 94: 6480-6483.

Marshall, C.G., Lessard, I.A., Park, I., and Wright, G.D. 1998. Glycopeptide antibiotic resistance genes in glycopeptide-producing organisms. Antimicrob. Agents Chemother. 42: 2215-2220.

Martone, W.J. 1998. Spread of vancomycin-resistant enterococci: why did it happen in the United States? Infect. Control Hosp. Epidemiol. 19: 539-545.

Ma, X.X., Ito, T., Tiensasitorn, C., Jamklang M., Chongtrakool, P., Boyle-Vavra, S., Daum, R.S. and Hiramatsu, K. 2002. Novel type of staphylococcal cassette chromosome *mec* identified in community-acquired methicillin-resistant *Staphylococcus aureus* strains. Antimicrob. Agents Chemother. 46: 1147-52.

McDonald, L.C., Rossiter, S., Mackinson, C., Wang, Y.Y., Johnson, S., Sullivan, M., Sokolow, R., DeBess, E., Gilbert, L., Benson, J.A., Hill, B., and Angulo, F.J. 2001. Quinupristin-dalfopristin-resistant *Enterococcus faecium* on chicken and in human stool specimens. N. Engl. J. Med. 345: 1155-1160.

McDougal, L.K., and Thornsberry, C. 1986. The role of beta-lactamase in staphylococcal resistance to penicillinase-resistant penicillins and cephalosporins. J. Clin. Microbiol. 23: 832-839.

McKessar, S.J., Berry, A.M., Bell, J.M., Turnidge, J.D., and Paton, J.C. 2000. Genetic characterization of *vanG*, a novel vancomycin resistance locus of *Enterococcus faecalis*. Antimicrob. Agents Chemother. 44: 3224-3228.

Mederski-Samoraj, B.D., and Murray, B.E. 1983. High-level resistance to gentamicin in clinical isolates of enterococci. J. Infect. Dis. 147: 751-757.

Miller, M.H., Wexler, M.A., and Steigbigel, N.H. 1978. Single and combination antibiotic therapy of *Staphylococcus aureus* experimental endocarditis: emergence of gentamicin-resistant mutants. Antimicrob. Agents Chemother. 14: 336-343.

Moellering, R.C., Linden, P.K., Reinhardt, J., Blumberg, E.A., Bompart, F., and Talbot, G.H. 1999. The efficacy and safety of quinupristin/dalfopristin for the treatment of infections caused by vancomycin-resistant *Enterococcus faecium*. Synercid Emergency-Use Study Group. J. Antimicrob. Chemother. 44: 251-261.

Monnet, D.L. 1998. Methicillin-resistant *Staphylococcus aureus* and its relationship to antimicrobial use: possible implications for control. Infect. Control Hosp. Epidemiol. 19: 552-559.

Monnet, D.L., and Frimodt-Moller, N. 2001. Antimicrobial-drug use and methicillin-resistant *Staphylococcus aureus*. Emerg. Infect. Dis. 7: 161-163.

Morris, J.G., Jr., Shay, D.K., Hebden, J.N., McCarter, R.J., Jr., Perdue, B.E., Jarvis, W., Johnson, J.A., Dowling, T.C., Polish, L.B., and Schwalbe, R.S. 1995. Enterococci resistant to multiple antimicrobial agents, including vancomycin. Establishment of endemicity in a university medical center. Ann. Intern. Med. 123: 250-259.

Morton, T.M., Johnston, J.L., Patterson, J., and Archer, G.L. 1995. Characterization of a conjugative staphylococcal mupirocin resistance plasmid. Antimicrob. Agents Chemother. 39: 1272-1280.

Mulligan, M.E., Murray-Leisure, K.A., Ribner, B.S., Standiford, H.C., John, J.F., Korvick, J.A., Kauffman, C.A., and Yu, V.L. 1993. Methicillin-resistant *Staphylococcus aureus*: a consensus review of the microbiology, pathogenesis, and epidemiology with implications for prevention and management. Am. J. Med. 94: 313-328.

Murray, B.E. 1990. The life and times of the Enterococcus. Clin. Microbiol. Rev. 3: 46-65.

Murray, B.E. 1992. Beta-lactamase-producing enterococci. Antimicrob. Agents Chemother. 36: 2355-2359.

Murray, B.E. 2000. Vancomycin-resistant enterococcal infections. N. Engl. J. Med. 342: 710-721.

National Nosocomial Infections Surveillance System. 2001. Semiannual Report: Aggregated data from the National Nosocomial Infections Surveillance System, December 2000. Public Health Service, U.S. Department of Health and Human Services.

Navarro, F., and Courvalin, P. 1994. Analysis of genes encoding D-alanine-D-alanine ligase-related enzymes in *Enterococcus casseliflavus* and *Enterococcus flavescens*. Antimicrob. Agents Chemother. 38: 1788-1793.

Ng, E.Y., Trucksis, M., and Hooper, D.C. 1996. Quinolone resistance mutations in topoisomerase IV: relationship to the *flqA* locus and genetic evidence that topoisomerase IV is the primary target and DNA gyrase is the secondary target of fluoroquinolones in *Staphylococcus aureus*. Antimicrob. Agents Chemother. 40: 1881-1888.

Noble, W.C., Virani, Z., and Cree, R.G. 1992. Co-transfer of vancomycin and other resistance genes from *Enterococcus faecalis* NCTC 12201 to *Staphylococcus aureus*. FEMS Microbiol. Lett. 72: 195-198.

Nord, C.E., Heimdahl, A., Kager, L., and Malmborg, A.S. 1984. The impact of different antimicrobial agents on the normal gastrointestinal microflora of humans. Rev. Infect. Dis. 6 Suppl. 1: S270-S275.

Ostrowsky, B.E., Trick, W.E., Sohn, A.H., Quirk, S.B., Holt, S., Carson, L.A., Hill, B.C., Arduino, M.J., Kuehnert, M.J., and Jarvis, W.R. 2001. Control of vancomycin-resistant enterococcus in health care facilities in a region. N. Engl. J. Med. 344: 1427-1433.

Pallares, R., Pujol, M., Pena, C., Ariza, J., Martin, R., and Gudiol, F. 1993. Cephalosporins as risk factor for nosocomial *Enterococcus faecalis* bacteremia. A matched case-control study. Arch Intern Med. 153: 1581-1586.

Panlilio, A.L., Culver, D.H., Gaynes, R.P., Banerjee, S., Henderson, T.S., Tolson, J.S., and Martone, W.J. 1992. Methicillin-resistant *Staphylococcus aureus* in U.S. hospitals, 1975- 1991. Infect. Control Hosp. Epidemiol. 13: 582-586.

Parker, M.T., and Hewitt, J.H. 1970. Methicillin resistance in *Staphylococcus aureus*. Lancet. 1: 800-804.

Patel, R., Piper, K., Cockerill, F.R., 3rd, Steckelberg, J.M., and Yousten, A.A. 2000. The biopesticide *Paenibacillus popilliae* has a vancomycin resistance gene cluster homologous to the enterococcal VanA vancomycin resistance gene cluster. Antimicrob. Agents Chemother. 44: 705-709.

Plorde, J.J., and Sherris, J.C. 1974. Staphylococcal resistance to antibiotics: origin, measurement, and epidemiology. Ann. N.Y. Acad. Sci. 236: 413-434.

Portillo, A., Ruiz-Larrea, F., Zarazaga, M., Alonso, A., Martinez, J.L., and Torres, C. 2000. Macrolide resistance genes in *Enterococcus* spp. Antimicrob. Agents Chemother. 44: 967-971.

Prystowsky, J., Siddiqui, F., Chosay, J., Shinabarger, D.L., Millichap, J., Peterson, L.R., and Noskin, G.A. 2001. Resistance to linezolid: characterization of mutations in rRNA and comparison of their occurrences in vancomycin-resistant enterococci. Antimicrob. Agents Chemother. 45: 2154-2156.

Quale, J., Landman, D., Saurina, G., Atwood, E., DiTore, V., and Patel, K. 1996. Manipulation of a hospital antimicrobial formulary to control an outbreak of vancomycin-resistant enterococci. Clin. Infect. Dis. 23: 1020-1025.

Reagan, D.R., Doebbeling, B.N., Pfaller, M.A., Sheetz, C.T., Houston, A.K., Hollis, R.J., and Wenzel, R.P. 1991. Elimination of coincident *Staphylococcus aureus* nasal and hand carriage with intranasal application of mupirocin calcium ointment. Ann. Intern. Med. 114: 101-106.

Report of a combined working party of the Hospital Infection Society and British Society for Antimicrobial Chemotherapy. 1990. Revised guidelines for the control of epidemic methicillin-resistant *Staphylococcus aureus*. J. Hosp. Infect. 16: 351-377.

Rice, L.B. 2001. Emergence of vancomycin-resistant enterococci. Emerg. Infect. Dis. 7: 183-187.

Rice, L.B., Carias, L.L., Donskey, C.L., and Rudin, S.D. 1998. Transferable, plasmid-mediated *vanB*-type glycopeptide resistance in *Enterococcus faecium*. Antimicrob. Agents Chemother. 42: 963-964.

Sahm, D.F., Marsilio, M.K., and Piazza, G. 1999. Antimicrobial resistance in key bloodstream bacterial isolates: electronic surveillance with the Surveillance Network Database—USA. Clin. Infect. Dis. 29: 259-263.

Sanford, M.D., Widmer, A.F., Bale, M.J., Jones, R.N., and Wenzel, R.P. 1994. Efficient detection and long-term persistence of the carriage of methicillin-resistant *Staphylococcus aureus*. Clin. Infect. Dis. 19: 1123-1128.

Saravolatz, L.D., Markowitz, N., Arking, L., Pohlod, D., and Fisher, E. 1982. Methicillin-resistant *Staphylococcus aureus*. Epidemiologic observations during a community-acquired outbreak. Ann. Intern. Med. 96: 11-16.

Schaberg, D.R., Culver, D.H., and Gaynes, R.P. 1991. Major trends in the microbial etiology of nosocomial infection. Am. J. Med. 91: 72S-75S.

Schmitz, F.J., Sadurski, R., Kray, A., Boos, M., Geisel, R., Kohrer, K., Verhoef, J., and Fluit, A.C. 2000. Prevalence of macrolide-resistance genes in *Staphylococcus aureus* and *Enterococcus faecium* isolates from 24 European university hospitals. J. Antimicrob. Chemother. 45: 891-894.

Schouten, M.A., Voss, A., Hoogkamp-Korstanje, J.A. and The European VRE Study Group 1999. Antimicrobial susceptibility patterns of enterococci causing infections in Europe. Antimicrob. Agents Chemother. 43: 2542-2546.

Schouten, M.A., Hoogkamp-Korstanje, J.A., Meis, J.F., Voss, A. and The European VRE Study Group. 2000. Prevalence of vancomycin resistant Enterococci in Europe. Eur. J. Clin. Microbiol. Infect. Dis. 19: 816-822.

Schwalbe, R.S., Stapleton, J.T., and Gilligan, P.H. 1987. Emergence of vancomycin resistance in coagulase-negative staphylococci. N. Engl. J. Med. 316: 927-931.

Sheretz, R.J., Reagan, D.R., Hampton, K.D., Robertson, K.L., Streed, S.A., Hoen, H.M., Thomas, R., and Gwaltney, J.M., Jr. 1996. A cloud adult: the *Staphylococcus aureus*-virus interaction revisited. Ann. Intern. Med. 124: 539-547.

Sherris, J.C. 1986. Problems in *in vitro* determination of antibiotic tolerance in clinical isolates. Antimicrob. Agents Chemother. 30: 633-637.

Sieradzki, K., and Tomasz, A. 1997. Inhibition of cell wall turnover and autolysis by vancomycin in a highly vancomycin-resistant mutant of *Staphylococcus aureus*. J. Bacteriol. 179: 2557-2566.

Sifaoui, F., Arthur, M., Rice, L., and Gutmann, L. 2001. Role of penicillin-binding protein 5 in expression of ampicillin resistance and peptidoglycan structure in *Enterococcus faecium*. Antimicrob. Agents Chemother. 45: 2594-2597.

Tally, F.P., and DeBruin, M.F. 2000. Development of daptomycin for gram-positive infections. J. Antimicrob. Chemother. 46: 523-526.

Tenover, F.C., Biddle, J.W., and Lancaster, M.V. 2001. Increasing resistance to vancomycin and other glycopeptides in *Staphylococcus aureus*. Emerg. Infect. Dis. 7: 327-332.

Tofte, R.W., Solliday, J.A., and Crossley, K.B. 1984. Susceptibilities of enterococci to twelve antibiotics. Antimicrob. Agents Chemother. 25: 532-533.

Tornieporth, N.G., Roberts, R.B., John, J., Hafner, A., and Riley, L.W. 1996. Risk factors associated with vancomycin-resistant *Enterococcus faecium* infection or colonization in 145 matched case patients and control patients. Clin. Infect. Dis. 23: 767-772.

Tsiodras, S., Gold, H.S., Sakoulas, G., Eliopoulos, G.M., Wennersten, C., Venkataraman, L., Moellering, R.C., and Ferraro, M.J. 2001. Linezolid resistance in a clinical isolate of *Staphylococcus aureus*. Lancet. 358: 207-208.

Uttley, A.H., Collins, C.H., Naidoo, J., and George, R.C. 1988. Vancomycin-resistant enterococci. Lancet. 1: 57-58.

Van der Auwera, P., Pensart, N., Korten, V., Murray, B.E., and Leclercq, R. 1996. Influence of oral glycopeptides on the fecal flora of human volunteers: selection of highly glycopeptide-resistant enterococci. J. Infect. Dis. 173: 1129-1136.

Vergis, E.N., Hayden, M.K., Chow, J.W., Snydman, D.R., Zervos, M.J., Linden, P.K., Wagener, M.M., Schmitt, B., and Muder, R.R. 2001. Determinants of vancomycin resistance and mortality rates in enterococcal bacteremia. a prospective multicenter study. Ann. Intern. Med. 135: 484-492.

Voladri, R.K., Tummuru, M.K., and Kernodle, D.S. 1996. Structure-function relationships among wild-type variants of *Staphylococcus aureus* beta-lactamase: importance of amino acids 128 and 216. J. Bacteriol. 178: 7248-7253.

von Eiff, C., Becker, K., Machka, K., Stammer, H., and Peters, G. 2001. Nasal carriage as a source of *Staphylococcus aureus* bacteremia. Study Group. N. Engl. J. Med. 344: 11-16.

Voss, A., Milatovic, D., Wallrauch-Schwarz, C., Rosdahl, V.T., and Braveny, I. 1994. Methicillin-resistant *Staphylococcus aureus* in Europe. Eur. J. Clin. Microbiol. Infect. Dis. 13: 50-55.

Walsh, C.T., Fisher, S.L., Park, I.S., Prahalad, M., and Wu, Z. 1996. Bacterial resistance to vancomycin: five genes and one missing hydrogen bond tell the story. Chem. Biol. 3: 21-28.

Wanger, A.R., and Murray, B.E. 1990. Comparison of enterococcal and staphylococcal beta-lactamase plasmids. J. Infect. Dis. 161: 54-58.

Watanakunakorn, C., and Patel, R. 1993. Comparison of patients with enterococcal bacteremia due to strains with and without high-level resistance to gentamicin. Clin. Infect. Dis. 17: 74-78.

Weber, D.J., and Rutala, W.A. 1997. Role of environmental contamination in the transmission of vancomycin- resistant enterococci. Infect. Control Hosp. Epidemiol. 18: 306-309.

Weinstein, M.R., Dedier, H., Brunton, J., Campbell, I., and Conly, J.M. 1999. Lack of efficacy of oral bacitracin plus doxycycline for the eradication of stool colonization with vancomycin-resistant *Enterococcus faecium*. Clin. Infect. Dis. 29: 361-366.

Wenzel, R.P., Reagan, D.R., Bertino, J.S., Jr., Baron, E.J., and Arias, K. 1998. Methicillin-resistant *Staphylococcus aureus* outbreak: a consensus panel's definition and management guidelines. Am. J. Infect. Control. 26: 102-110.

Werner, G., Klare, I., Heier, H., Hinz, K.H., Bohme, G., Wendt, M., and Witte, W. 2000. Quinupristin/dalfopristin-resistant enterococci of the *satA* (*vatD*) and *satG* (*vatE*) genotypes from different ecological origins in Germany. Microb. Drug Resist. 6: 37-47.

Wong, M.T., Kauffman, C.A., Standiford, H.C., Linden, P., Fort, G., Fuchs, H.J., Porter, S.B., and Wenzel, R.P. 2001. Effective suppression of vancomycin-resistant *Enterococcus* species in asymptomatic gastrointestinal carriers by a novel glycolipodepsipeptide, ramoplanin. Clin. Infect. Dis. 33: 1476-1482.

Wu, S.W., de Lencastre, H., and Tomasz, A. 2001. Recruitment of the *mecA* gene homologue of *Staphylococcus sciuri* into a resistance determinant and expression of the resistant phenotype in *Staphylococcus aureus*. J. Bacteriol. 183: 2417-2424.

Yuk, J.H., Dignani, M.C., Harris, R.L., Bradshaw, M.W., and Williams, T.W., Jr. 1991. Minocycline as an alternative anti- staphylococcal agent. Rev. Infect. Dis. 13: 1023-1024.

From: *Multiple Drug Resistant Bacteria*
Edited by: Carlos F. Amábile-Cuevas

Chapter 7

Horizontal Gene Transfer and the Selection of Antibiotic Resistance

Jack A. Heinemann and
Mark W. Silby

Abstract

Gene transfer between organisms is usually studied from the view of how the transferred genes benefit the organism to which they have transferred. Indeed, many studies of horizontal (lateral) gene transfer are really descriptions of organisms that have survived because of, or despite, past gene transfers. Other studies focus on the biochemical mechanisms of gene transfer. Few studies are about how horizontal gene transfer evolved and is evolving. The conclusions of those studies are emphasized here. Antibiotic use in medicine and agriculture has made an important contribution to our understanding of gene transfer. We will discuss how understanding the evolution of horizontal gene transfer could help in the search for a new generation of agents to treat infectious diseases.

Introduction

Modern antimicrobial agents all have one activity in common: they interrupt the reproduction of genes that reproduce synchronously with organisms. In the case of bacteria, those genes are found almost universally on chromosomes. Other heritable states and genes (Cogoni and Macino, 2000; Heinemann and Roughan, 2000; Strohman, 1997; Weld and Heinemann, 2002) that can reproduce independently of host reproduction, for example by horizontal gene transfer (HGT), are inconsistently affected by antimicrobial agents. It is perhaps this insight that best underscores requirements for the next generation of chemotherapies to treat infectious diseases. Existing agents were screened for both low toxicity to patients and maximum inhibition of microbes. New agents must still be screened for low toxicity to patients, but also developed to cure disease without invoking resistance (Heinemann, 1999; 2001). Whereas biochemistry and physiology have been excellent guides for identifying agents with the former two qualities, it will be evolutionary theory and gene ecology that guide our quest for agents with the latter qualities.

The literature is replete with evidence of HGT. The evidence is provided for: mechanisms of gene transfer that know no phylogenetic boundaries (de la Cruz and Davies, 2000; Ferguson and Heinemann, 2002); bioinformatic evidence of carcases of "foreign" genes within genomes (Doolittle, 1999b; Gogarten and Olendzenski, 1999; Ochman *et al.*, 2000); and, more importantly, the identification of properties of genes that can only be attributed to selection acting upon them independently of the host (Cooper and Heinemann, 2000; Denamur *et al.*, 2000; Jain et al., 1999; Kobayashi, 1998; Kolstø, 1997; Lawrence, 1997). So whereas, in retrospect, HGT appears to have provided an explanation for both the extent and pace of resistance evolution, it has not significantly influenced approaches to drug discovery (Heinemann, 2001). We will describe how insights into the way HGT influences the evolution of both genes and genotypes (Heinemann, 2000) might be translated into the mechanics of drug discovery.

"We need to look for, and try to understand, those features of structure and function of genes that bear on their survival and spread as independent agents within the global superorganism" (Doolittle, 1999a).

Is antibiotic resistance a phenomenon of natural selection tempering the reproduction of bacteria or, instead, a phenomenon of natural selection tempering the reproduction of genes? There are at least two phases in the evolution of antibiotic-resistant bacteria. The first phase, and the one most relevant to the useful life of anti-infective agents, is only indirectly related to the differential success of resistant bacteria in the presence of antibiotics. The evolution of genes, like antibiotic resistance, is driven by structural and functional attributes that bear on their spread between organisms (Heinemann, 2001). This is surprising because antibiotic resistance *per se* is not involved in HGT. To properly appreciate this conclusion requires that old views of the relationship between genes and organisms, genotypes and phenotypes, be reconsidered. The second phase of resistance evolution is consistent with what Levin and Bergstrom might call "informal (verbal)" evolutionary theories of prokaryotic evolution (Levin and Bergstrom, 2000), and involves the spread of recombinant organisms whose reproduction is a function of selection acting on the organismal phenotype. Phase two has been the traditional focus of drug designers.

"We can regard the gene as an organ in the cell, just as the heart, pancreas, or femur is an organ in the body as a whole" (Haldane, 1941).

To properly address phase one evolution requires discarding some familiar views of the gene. Is the gene a metaphorical organ, seen only by natural selection through the gene's function within the cell? Or can the gene sometimes be thought of as an independent agent, related to the cell in which it is sometimes found by a combination of historical contingency, function and as a result of its own evolution governed in part by its ability to reproduce independently of the cell? The Haldane metaphor for genes captures how genes are informally thought about by many biologists. Nevertheless, that view of genes has not inspired new insights into how anti-infective agents might be designed (Heinemann, 2001).

Genomes may sometimes evolve as organs of cellular organisms and sometimes as agents with a separate relationship to natural selection. Knowing when they are organs and when they are agents with an independent responsiveness to natural selection bears on predictions of gene function ranging from the risk of genetically modified organisms through the design of antimicrobial agents to bioinformatics. The degree to which a genome has evolved with the organism in which it is found corresponds with the confidence in making phylogenetic associations. The degree to which genomes (or constituent genes) defy

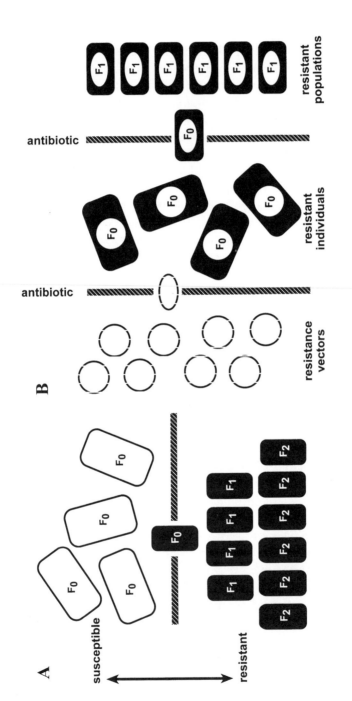

Figure 1. How antibiotics select antibiotic-resistance. (A) Canonical model of antibiotic-resistance evolution. Rare pre-existing variants (solid rectangles) within larger populations of antibiotic-susceptible bacteria (open rectangles) continue to produce offspring following the introduction of an antibiotic into the environment. Susceptible bacteria produce no more generations beyond the initial F_0. (B) The canonical model does not explain the near universal occurrence of resistance genes initially and sometimes persistently on vectors (open circles and ovals) that reproduce by horizontal gene transfer. Some vectors (open ovals) acquire resistance genes. When these enter susceptible bacteria prior to the introduction of antibiotics, they convert genotypically susceptible bacteria (open rectangles) into resistant (solid rectangles). These recombinants then amplify in the environment.

phylogeny undermine associations at the heart of bioinformatic theory (Martin, 1999).

When an antibiotic resistance gene contributes to the survival and subsequent reproduction of a bacterium (phase two), the resistance gene is acting as an organ of the organism (Figure 1A). The gene itself is reproducing as a consequence of the reproduction of the host. The resistance gene could be on a plasmid, virus or chromosome to achieve the same effect. But in possibly all clinically relevant microbes, the genes (or functionally significant constituent nucleotide sequences (Fitch, 2000)) conferring resistance are newer to the organism than many other genes (Figure 1B). So even chromosomally encoded resistances, such as penicillin resistance due to alterations of pencillin-binding proteins (Spratt, 1994), can be assembled by HGT. If resistance evolution were solely, even primarily, the function of selection acting on the overall phenotypes of organisms, then the resistant pathogens that are circulating through hospitals should be direct descendants of progenitor strains that acquired resistance to the first generation of antimicrobial agents to which they were genotypically susceptible. A record of resistance genes should be found in their genomes and that record should link together an unbroken chain of resistances to each antimicrobial agent since their clinical introductions. But the spread of multiple resistance is not systematic and clonal but *ad hoc* and bricolage. Resistance phenotypes arise from the conversion of genes reproducing by HGT into genes that also reproduce synchronously with organisms.

"Taken together, (the new data) threaten to throw the very concept of 'the gene'—either as a unit of structure or as a unit of function—into blatant disarray" (Keller, 2000).

The idea that genes on plasmids, transposons and other vectors are there because they adapt bacteria to environments with antibiotics begs the question: how do antibiotics select for resistance genes on such vectors to begin with (Figure 1B)? Genes can have their own relationship to evolution through selection that acts on them as agents of reproduction rather than indirectly through their contribution to the reproduction of the organism (Heinemann and Roughan, 2000; Souza and Eguiarte, 1997). This view is often confused with the "Selfish DNA" theory, but is not entirely consistent with that theory (Box 1).

Box 1

"The selfish DNA theory...argued that plasmids and transposable elements should be viewed as genetic parasites, whose sometimes beneficial effects on the long-term evolvability of prokaryotic hosts are coincidental" (Doolittle, 1999a).

The Selfish DNA theory argued that the evolutionary success of an organism does not imply the value of all its inheritable parts. Many have, and still do, labor under the adaptationist assumption that phenotypes and the genes that cause them are the product of selection (*e.g.,* Heinemann, 1993). Are antibiotic resistance genes and their vectors, plasmids and transposable-type elements, selfish DNA?

Selfishness describes an outcome (the inclusion within genomes of genes that have no or a deleterious effect on organismal fitness), not an evolutionary or biological process. The difficulty with selfish DNA as a way to view antibiotic resistance is that the 'theory' attempts to reconcile the evolution of elements that accumulate in fundamentally different ways, and are irreconcilable by the precepts of selfishness. Selfish DNA is thought to include both genetic agents that respond to natural selection and genetic agents that reproduce in response to selection acting on the organism in which they are found. For example, it seeks to explain both junk DNA (Doolittle and Sapienza, 1980; Orgel and Crick, 1980), which accumulates within genomes, and elements like plasmids and viruses that accumulate through reproduction separate from the host, by HGT. Genetic phenomena are not always the result or cause of evolution and the ultimate proliferation of repetitive sequences cannot be separated from the reproduction of the organism in which they proliferate. The Selfish DNA theory only applies to genes reproducing within an organism when the fate of the gene and organism are inseparable.

We know of only one empirical example of selfish DNA that meets the test (Orgel and Crick, 1980) for it, and in that case the important qualities were the ability to reproduce by HGT and to kill the host (Figure 3), not increase within a genome. Other elements that simply had the ability to spread by HGT also failed to increase in number as selfish elements should (Condit, 1990). Thus, antibiotic resistance evolution appears to fulfil the conditions of selfishness at best only sometimes (possibly in phase one), and rigorously it has never been shown to fit the conditions of selfishness.

Box 1, Continued

Even though the Selfish DNA view is consistent in parts with what is being presented here, we have taken an adaptationist view because we accord the gene-selection relationship the same agency as the organism-selection relationship.

So whereas the genes may have since been captured by chromosomes for their value to the organism (phase two evolution) or because of their latent selfish qualities (Kobayashi, 1998; Kusano *et al.*, 1995), phase one evolution probably explains their HGT origins (especially the recent incursion of antibiotic resistance genes into clinically relevant pathogens). Post-segregational killing genes (PSK), for example, attack other infectious elements, such as competing plasmids and viruses, but do not necessarily increase the absolute rate of reproduction of the vector (Box 2). In this way, the genes are not selfish.

Inconsistent with canonical Selfish DNA views (Dawkins, 1989), the relationship between genes and selection has contextual boundaries rather than different effects at different biological scales of complexity. The same gene that can at times negotiate its relationship to evolution directly, can at other times have its relationship to evolution be conditioned through the host. Recognising the two phases, and then identifying the "principles (that) must govern the distribution of genes" (Martin, 1999) between the phases at any given time, are the challenges ahead in attempts to design the evolution of anti-infective agents.

How do Genes Gain Direct Access to Natural Selection?

The ability to reproduce is a prerequisite for evolution by natural selection. If two reproducing entities can do so independently of one another, then the reproduction of one entity can potentially impact on the other.

Antibiotics create environments in which the reproduction of some genes occurs independently of the reproduction of other genes in an organism's genome (Figure 2). We have identified nine illustrative environments where this occurs (Cooper and Heinemann, 2000; Ferguson *et al.*, 2000, 2002; Heinemann, 1999). In contrast, the genes that only reproduce synchronously with the organism are evolving at a

NICHES FOR GENE TRANSFER CREATED BY ANTIBIOTICS

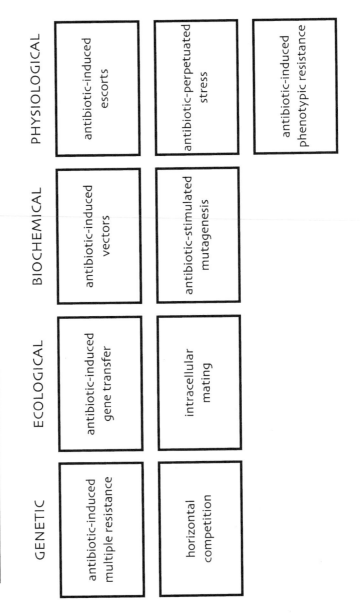

GENETIC	ECOLOGICAL	BIOCHEMICAL	PHYSIOLOGICAL
antibiotic-induced multiple resistance	antibiotic-induced gene transfer	antibiotic-induced vectors	antibiotic-induced escorts
horizontal competition	intracellular mating	antibiotic-stimulated mutagenesis	antibiotic-perpetuated stress
			antibiotic-induced phenotypic resistance

Figure 2. Antibiotics create special niches for HGT. Antibiotics are usually discussed from the view of how they differ from one another—chemically, by target specificity, and by activity range. What they have in common may be a clue to how to design different types of infection control agents. What all these agents have in common is that they prevent the reproduction of chromosomes. They also have in common the ability to create genetic, ecological, biochemical and physiological niches for gene transfer (Heinemann, 1999; Heinemann *et al.*, 2000).

For example, one antibiotic can select for resistance to several antibiotics because HGT vectors often carry more than one resistance gene (Salyers and Amábile-Cuevas, 1997). One antibiotic can induce the expression of efflux pumps effective against multiple antibiotics. Even in the case of cell-wall damaging agents like β-lactam antibiotics, in some environments the effect of the agent is to increase HGT (Heinemann, 1999). Bacteria that invade human cells are protected from antibiotics and there can exchange resistance genes even with non-invasive bacteria (Ferguson *et al.*, 2002). The genes themselves may have the ability to drive their evolution independently of the benefit of the gene to the bacterium (Cooper and Heinemann, 2000).

rate proportional to the organism as a whole, as a result of natural selection acting on overall phenotype of the organism. For operational purposes, we define collections of these genes as chromosomal even if the chromosomes themselves are mosaics of genes distributed across phases one and two (Heinemann, 2000).

Genes with other reproductive options, for examples those on conjugative plasmids of bacteria, viruses, and other vectors, such as the *cis*-acting signal sequences in the DNA of some naturally competent bacteria, exist in a different evolutionary space from chromosomes (Heinemann and Roughan, 2000). This space is defined by the ecology of genes rather than the resource requirements of organisms. First, HGT occurs between organisms that can no longer reproduce themselves or their chromosomal genes (*i.e.*, dead), between species (which operationally define the barriers to chromosomal genes) and potentially between dead members of one species and the live members of another. Second, cellular organisms reproduce at a rate that is ultimately limited by sequestering enough resources to re-create the organism, at least to the sophistication of a cell. Genes that reproduce infectiously, for example by HGT, are only limited by time in this activity— that is, as long as organisms already exist and genes can jump between them. Time-limited reproduction is a realistic possibility, because the world is like an intact biofilm, or superorganism (Dixon, 1994; Whitman *et al.*, 1998). HGT allows genes to evolve not just *in* parallel with organisms, but parallel *to* organisms.

Antibiotics prevent the reproduction of chromosomal genes in as much as they inhibit or prevent the reproduction of bacteria. But most antibiotics, at least under some conditions, fail to prevent HGT. Others

Box 2

"Did mechanisms of programmed cell death in eukaryotes and prokaryotes evolve from common antecedents? (It appears) safe to say that similar purposes are served" (Yarmolinsky, 1995).

The idea that PSK genes are effective equivalents of those that cause apoptosis in multicellular organisms (Yarmolinsky, 1995) is intriguing, but has not proved a useful heuristic for understanding the evolution of such genes either in multicellular organisms or in prokaryotes. Like the selfish DNA hypotheses, the apoptosis view seeks to find a role for deleterious, but nevertheless successful, genes.

Apoptosis and antibiotics, however, might be useful to prokaryotes, especially in biofilms, and thus may sometimes be the end product of phase two evolution. Antibiotics may have important roles in developing or maintaining community structure (de Lorenzo and Aguilar, 1984; Kell *et al.*, 1995). Colicins and microcins, antibiotic compounds common to enterobacteria of mammalian flora for example, could regulate succession of microbial communities in this environment. Likewise, human use of antibiotics may influence the powerful dynamics of gene-gene competitions; some resistance genotypes may arise and disappear as a result (Westh *et al.*, 1995). The role of antibiotics may be communicative in nature, like pheromones secreted by yeast (Kell *et al.*, 1995). When humans artificially saturate environments with particular classes of antibiotics, they may favor the colonization or hegemony of the microbial species that would employ those same or similar antibiotics to obtain or protect the niche. Those organisms that utilize a particular antibiotic of course also maintain a state of resistance to that antibiotic. Thus, human application engineers a macroscopic bias on microbial communities, favoring the establishment of communities bonded through antibiotics (de Lorenzo and Aguilar, 1984; Neu, 1992).

Could the use of antibiotics create a niche in hospitals for species uncompetitive in the absence of antibiotics? Kehoe et al. (Kehoe *et al.*, 1996) have commented on the noticeable decline in incidence and severity of some group A streptococcal diseases beginning prior to the introduction of antibiotic therapies and the sudden and dramatic reappearance of group A streptococcal diseases in the 1980s. Could the ecological conditions that favored the decline of virulent group A streptococci earlier in the century have been neutralized or reversed by the use of antibiotics?

Box 2, Continued

Since the clinical introduction of antibiotics, there has been a succession in species that most frequently cause nosocomial infections (Emori and Gaynes, 1993; Neu, 1992; Spera and Farber, 1992; Swartz, 1994), suggesting that perhaps antibiotics favored species that had an intrinsic capacity to more quickly develop resistance or whose life style was advantaged in some other way by human application of antibiotics (Garrett, 1994).

---

can increase the relative rate of reproduction by HGT (Heinemann, 1999; Heinemann *et al.*, 2000). Thus, antibiotic resistance genes can evolve on HGT vectors in the presence of antibiotics. But why are resistance genes on HGT vectors in the first place? Or why have they not always been on HGT vectors (Eberhard, 1989)? The 'competition model' was introduced as a starting point for engaging these fundamental biological questions.

"Could physical environment and ecology be as strong a determinant of a genome's composition as phylogeny?" (Doolittle, 1999b).

The Competition Model

The mutually exclusive reproduction of two genetic units is the essence of the 'competition model' (Heinemann, 1998; Heinemann and Roughan, 2000). If entities can compete for reproductive success, then they are being subject to a selection for the better competitor in that particular environment. If competition between genes can be detected, even in the absence of an overall increase in the reproduction of the competitors, then that is *prima facie* evidence of natural selection acting on the gene.

Like other genes common to plasmids, such as the post-segregational killing genes (PSK) genes (Gerdes *et al.*, 1986; Naito *et al.*, 1995), antibiotic resistance genes could confer reproductive advantages in some environments upon vectors that reproduce by HGT (Cooper and Heinemann, 2000). PSK genes are any combination of genes that simultaneously produce a toxic effect on the host and suppress the toxic effect (Figure 3). Indeed, there is reason to believe that antibiotic resistance genes are PSK genes and thus have evolved in the same way (Heinemann, 1998). Others view the relationship of PSK genes to the host as the defining characteristic of their evolution (*e.g.*, Box 2). This may be true for phase two evolution, but not phase one.

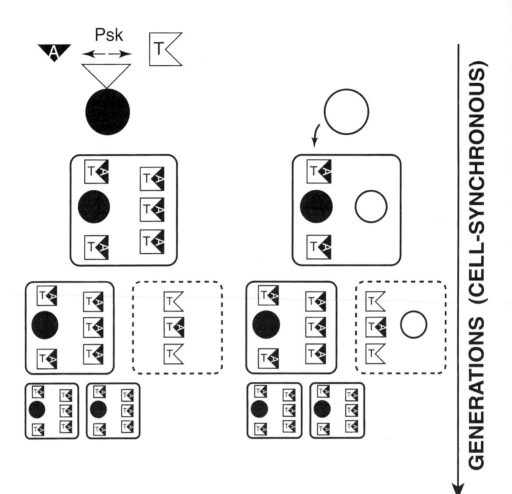

Figure 3. Structural and functional features of PSK in phase one and phase two evolution. Plasmids (circles) encoding post-segregational killing (Psk) systems (solid circles) produce toxin (pentagon) and antidote (triangle) molecules. If the plasmid mis-segregates during cell-synchronous reproduction, the plasmid-less daughter (dashed-line) inherits the stable toxin and soon loses the unstable antidote, leading to cell death. The other daughter (solid line) continues to reproduce. Thus, PSK plasmids are very "stable" and can develop associations for phase two evolution. In the competition model, plasmids without Psk (open circles) are driven from populations of bacteria when Psk-bearing plasmids enter the same host, forcing the former plasmid into daughters lacking the gene for the antidote molecules. Thus, plasmids with PSK systems are selected in phase one evolution.

The structural and functional attributes of PSK (Figure 3) are independent of the benefits such genes might provide the organismal host in the presence of antibiotics or other lethal agents (Naito *et al.*, 1995). The advantage PSK genes confer upon the HGT vector are even more important than the cost to organismal hosts for carrying the genes (Cooper and Heinemann, submitted Cooper and Heinemann, 2000).

PSK genes attack other infectious elements, for example, competing plasmids and viruses, but do not necessarily increase the absolute rate of reproduction of the vector. PSK genes were found to be significant disadvantages to vectors that were forced to reproduce at the rate of cell division (Cooper and Heinemann, 2000; Heinemann, 1998). Only when PSK was coupled to HGT did the vectors bearing PSK genes demonstrate competitiveness with vectors that did not have such genes.

The PSK method of attack is to kill cellular offspring that lose the genes. If a bacterium is infected by an invading virus or an incompatible plasmid, the PSK genes kill the bacterium along with the invading horizontally mobile element. In doing so, the PSK-bearing vector did not benefit with an immediate increase in reproduction, but it did eliminate a competitor.

Antibiotic resistance genes are functional PSK genes in the presence of antibiotics. This is because when a bacterium bearing a plasmid with a resistance gene is infected by an incompatible plasmid without the gene, the daughter inheriting the invader is killed by the antibiotic. Again, the resistance plasmid does not immediately reproduce more by killing the host of the competing plasmid, but it does eliminate the competitor. These models of evolution invoke a 'within-host' selection. Reminiscent of the old Batesonian contention that internal forces of selection are more important than external environments (Bateson, 1992; Heinemann, 1993), within-host selection predicts that PSK will evolve despite a significant cost to the host, and no immediate reproductive benefit to the vector.

PSK genes evolve by HGT, at least some of the time. They also create spectacular phenotypes, like antibiotic resistance and selective cell killing (*i.e.*, apoptosis) due to their biochemical activities. However, these phenotypes are only indirectly related to how PSK genes, like antibiotic resistance, converted from chromosomal to horizontally transferred genes. Selection acting on organisms with these genes may in time have found some use for them, but that is not an explanation for how the genes came to evolve on horizontally mobile elements.

The Different Predictions of the Competition Model

The competition model predicts that drugs that do not kill bacteria will not select for resistance genes on horizontally mobile elements. To some, this may seem trivial and immaterial because they would expect resistance to not evolve at all if the drug is not toxic. However, killing bacteria is not the only way to treat disease. It has been the easiest and most obvious way, but not necessarily the only way (Alksne and Projan, 2000; Highlander and Weinstock, 1992).

As argued elsewhere (Heinemann, 2001), the competition model offers some insights into how drugs that treat infectious diseases could be developed. These drugs may not immediately replace antibiotics. For acute cases, or when diagnosis technology is too slow, traditional antibiotics may remain the treatment of choice. For all other cases, drugs that prevent disease without killing microbes could be expected to accrue the same benefits as antibiotics without eliciting the cost of resistance.

PSK genes evolve on HGT vectors because they can be used to kill hosts of competing vectors. Although it is not the clinical intent to introduce antibiotics to engineer changes in gene vectors, antibiotics have effected that outcome. In contrast, drugs that cannot be used to resolve competitions at the gene level should not cause resistance genes to evolve by HGT and should delay or prevent bacterial drug resistance phenotypes.

The assumption of the competition model is that the benefits of virulence are not sufficient to overcome the stability of non-disease causing microbial communities. This remains to be shown. However, there is reason for optimism. Many infections arise because of disruptions in the benign microbial community (*e.g.*, Berg, 1995), not because of selection of virulence.

There is already the hope of new anti-infection agents near to development. Understanding the regulation of virulence phenotypes might produce avenues for microarray technology and proteomics to contribute to the development of more anti-infective, but "pro"-, biotics.

Some are targeting the vectors themselves (Amábile-Cuevas *et al.*, 1995). This approach has its dangers, but may be just brash enough to work.

Acknowledgements

JAH thanks the American Society for Microbiology for their contribution to his visit to LUSARA (Mexico City), where the content of this chapter was discussed with the Editor, and the University of Canterbury for grant U6333. Both authors wish to express their appreciation to T.F. Cooper for hours of stimulating conversation and contribution to results summarized herein.

References

Alksne, L.E. and Projan, S.J. 2000. Bacterial virulence as a target for antimicrobial chemotherapy. Curr. Opin. Biotech. 11: 625-636.

Amábile-Cuevas, C.F., Cárdenas-García, M. and Ludgar, M. 1995. Antibiotic Resistance. Amer. Sci. 83: 320-329.

Bateson, W. 1992. Materials for the study of variation: treated with especial regard to discontinuity in the origin of species, 2nd Edition, P.M. Mabee and K. Fitzhugh, eds. The Johns Hopkins University Press, Baltimore (originally published in 1894)).

Berg, R.D. 1995. Bacterial translocation from the gastrointestinal tract. Trends Microbiol. 3: 149-154.

Cogoni, C. and Macino, G. 2000. Post-transcriptional gene silencing across kingdoms. Curr. Opin. Genet. Develop. 10: 638-643.

Condit, R. 1990. The evolution of transposable elements: conditions for establishment in bacterial populations. Evol. 44: 347-359.

Cooper, T.F. and Heinemann, J.A. 2000. Postsegregational killing does not increase plasmid stability but acts to mediate the exclusion of competing plasmids. Proc. Natl. Acad. Sci. USA 97: 12543-12648.

Dawkins, R. 1989. The selfish gene, 2nd Edition. Oxford University Press, Oxford.

de la Cruz, F. and Davies, J. 2000. Horizontal gene transfer and the origin of species: lessons from bacteria. Trends Microbiol. 8: 128-133.

de Lorenzo, V. and Aguilar, A. 1984. Antibiotics from gram-negative bacteria: do they play a role in microbial ecology? Trends Biochem. Sci. 266:

Denamur, E., Lecointre, G., Darlu, P., Tenaillon, O., Acquviva, C., Sayada, C., Sunjevaric, I., Rothstein, R., Elion, J., Taddei, F., Radman, M. and Matic, I. 2000. Evolutionary implications of the frequent horizontal transfer of mismatch repair genes. Cell 103: 711-721.

Dixon, B. 1994. Power unseen: how microbes rule the world. W.H. Freeman, Oxford.

Doolittle, W.F. 1999a. Lateral genomics. Trends Biochem. Sci. 24: M5-M8

Doolittle, W.F. 1999b. Phylogenetic classification and the universal tree (taxonomies based on molecular sequences). Science 284: 2124-2130.

Doolittle, W.F. and Sapienza, C. 1980. Selfish genes, the phenotype paradigm and genome evolution. Nature 284: 601-603.

Eberhard, W.G. 1989. Why do bacterial plasmids carry some genes and not others? Plasmid 21: 167-174.

Emori, T.G. and Gaynes, R.P. 1993. An overview of nosocomial infections, including the role of the microbiology laboratory. Clin. Microbiol. Rev. 6: 428-442.

Ferguson, G.C. and Heinemann, J.A. 2002. Recent history of trans-kingdom conjugation. In: Horizontal Gene Transfer, 2nd edition. C. I. Kado and M. Syvanen, eds. Harcourts, London. p. 3-17.

Ferguson, G.C., Heinemann, J.A. and Kennedy, M.A. 2002. Gene transfer between *Salmonella enterica* serovar Typhimurium inside epithelial cells. J. Bacteriol. 184: 2235-2242.

Fitch, W.M. 2000. Homology a personal view on some of the problems. Trends Genet. 16: 227-231.

Garrett, L. 1994. The coming plague: newly emerging diseases in a world out of balance. Farrar, Straus and Giroux, New York.

Gerdes, K., Rasmussen, P.B. and Molin, S. 1986. Unique type of plasmid maintenance function: postsegregational killing of plasmid-free cells. Proc. Natl. Acad. Sci. USA 83: 3116-3120.

Gogarten, J.P. and Olendzenski, L. 1999. Orthologs, paralogs and genome comparisons. Curr. Opin. Genet. Develop. 9: 630-636.

Haldane, J.B.S. 1941. New Paths in Genetics. George Allen and Unwin, London.

Heinemann, J.A. 1993. Bateson and peacocks' tails. Nature 363: 308.

Heinemann, J.A. 1998. Looking sideways at the evolution of replicons. In: Horizontal Gene Transfer. C.I. Kado and M. Syvanen, eds. International Thomson Publishing, London. p. 11-24.

Heinemann, J.A. 1999. How antibiotics cause antibiotic resistance. Drug Dis. Today 4: 72-79.

Heinemann, J.A. 2000. Horizontal transfer of genes between microorganisms. In: Encyclopedia of Microbiology. J. Lederberg, ed. Academic Press, San Diego. p. 698-706.

Heinemann, J.A. 2001. Can smart bullets penetrate magic bullet proof vests? Drug Dis. Today 6: 875-878.

Heinemann, J.A., Ankenbauer, R.G. and Amábile-Cuevas, C.F. 2000. Do antibiotics maintain antibiotic resistance? Drug Dis. Today 5: 195-204.

Heinemann, J.A. and Roughan, P.D. 2000. New hypotheses on the material nature of horizontally transferred genes. Ann. New York Acad. Sci. 906: 169-186.

Highlander, S.K. and Weinstock, G.M. 1992. Bacterial virulence factors as targets for chemotherapy. In: Emerging targets in antibacterial and antifungal chemotherapy. J. Sutcliffe and N.H. Georgopapadakou, eds. Chapman and Hall, New York. p. 323-346.

Jain, R., Rivera, M.C. and Lake, J.A. 1999. Horizontal gene transfer among genomes: the complexity hypothesis. Proc. Natl. Acad. Sci. USA 96: 3801-3806.

Kehoe, M. A., Kapur, V., Whatmore, A.M. and Musser, J.M. 1996. Horizontal gene transfer among group A streptococci: implications for pathogenesis and epidemiology. Trends Microbiol. 4: 436-443.

Kell, D. B., Kaprelyants, A.S. and Grafen, A. 1995. Pheromones, social behaviour and the functions of secondary metabolism in bacteria. Trends Ecol. Evol. 10: 126-129.

Keller, E.F. 2000. The century of the gene. Harvard University Press, Cambridge.

Kobayashi, I. 1998. Selfishness and death: raison d'être of restriction, recombination and mitochondria. Trends Genet. 14: 368-374.

Kolstø, A. 1997. Dynamic bacterial genome organization. Mol. Microbiol. 24: 241-248.

Kusano, K., Naito, T., Handa, N., and Kobayashi, I. 1995. Restriction-modification systems as genomic parasites in competition for specific sequences. Proc. Natl. Acad. Sci. USA 92: 11095-11099.

Lawrence, J.G. 1997. Selfish operons and speciation by gene transfer. Trends Microbiol. 5: 355-359.

Levin, B.R. and Bergstrom, C.T. 2000. Bacteria are different: observations, interpretations, speculations, and opinions about the mechanisms of adaptive evolution in prokaryotes. Proc. Natl. Acad. Sci. USA 97: 6981-6985.

Martin, W. 1999. Mosaic bacterial chromosomes: a challenge en route to a tree of genomes. BioEssays 21: 99-104.

Naito, T., Kusano, K. and Kobayashi, I. 1995. Selfish behavior of restriction-modification systems. Science 267: 897-899.

Neu, H.C. 1992. The crisis in antibiotic resistance. Science 257: 1064-1073.

Ochman, H., Lawrence, J.G. and Groisman, E.A. 2000. Lateral gene transfer and the nature of bacterial innovation. Nature 405: 299-304.

Orgel, L.E. and Crick, F.H.C. 1980. Selfish DNA: the ultimate parasite. Nature 284: 604-607.

Salyers, A.A. and Amábile-Cuevas, C.F. 1997. Why are antibiotic resistance genes so resistant to elimination? Antimicrob. Agents Chemother. 41: 2321-2325.

Souza, V. and Eguiarte, L.E. 1997. Bacteria gone native vs. bacteria gone awry?: plasmid transfer and bacterial evolution. Proc. Natl. Acad. Sci. USA 94: 5501-5503.

Spera, R.V., Jr. and Farber, B.F. 1992. Multiply-Resistant *Enterococcus faecium*. The nosocomial pathogen of the 1990s. J. Am. Med. Asoc. 268: 2563-2564.

Spratt, B.G. 1994. Resistance to antibiotics mediated by target alterations. Science 264: 388-393.

Strohman, R.C. 1997. The coming Kuhnian revolution in biology. Nature Biotech. 15: 194-200.

Swartz, M. N. 1994. Hospital-acquired infections: diseases with increasingly limited therapies. Proc. Natl. Acad. Sci. USA 91: 2420-2427.

Weld, R. and Heinemann, J.A. 2002. Horizontal transfer of proteins between species: part of the big picture or just a genetic vignette? In: Horizontal Gene Transfer, 2nd edition. C.I. Kado and M. Syvanen, eds. Harcourts, London. p51-62. .

Westh, H., Hougaard, D.M., Vuust, J. and Rosdahl, V.T. 1995. Prevalence of *erm* gene classes in erythromycin-resistant *Straphylococcus aureus* strains isolated between 1959 and 1988. Antimicrob. Agents Chemother. 39: 369-373.

Whitman, W.B., Coleman, D.C. and Wiebe, W.J. 1998. Prokaryotes: the unseen majority. Proc. Natl. Acad. Sci. USA 95: 6578-6583.

Yarmolinsky, M. B. 1995. Programmed cell death in bacterial populations. Science 267: 836-837.

Index